# Medical Ethics and the Elderly
# Second Edition

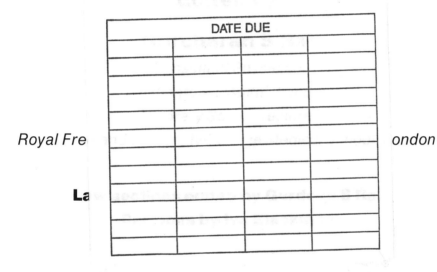

DATE DUE

*Royal Fre* *ondon*

**La**

'cliffe Medi
ord • Sa r

**Radcliffe Publishing Ltd**
18 Marcham Road
Abingdon
Oxon OX14 1AA
United Kingdom

**www.radcliffe-oxford.com**
Electronic catalogue and worldwide online ordering.

---

British Library Cataloguing in Publication Data

A catalogue record for this book is available from the British Library.

ISBN 1 85775 851X

Typeset by Aarontype Ltd, Easton, Bristol
Printed and bound by TJ International Ltd, Padstow, Cornwall

# Contents

# Foreword

The first edition of *Medical Ethics and the Elderly*, which appeared in 1999, was a landmark publication. Never before had practising clinicians in the field of geriatric medicine directed their attention so specifically to the everyday ethical problems that they face in clinical practice. The second edition is most welcome. As practising clinicians it often seems that we are making as many ethical decisions as clinical ones. We are all aware that these decisions require a considerable amount of expertise and skill. Applied medical ethics is a core competency of anyone practising within this field. Although there seems to be a growing ethics industry, very few available textbooks on medical ethics focus specifically on the problems of the older patient.

This book is characterised by incisive concise contributions that are directed at the central problems of clinical practice. The authors have an impressive range of experience, and their clinical acumen illuminates their ethical reasoning. The fact that a second edition has been necessary within three or four years of the first publication indicates not only that this is a growing and important field, but also that this book has been valued and used by many within the profession (including myself).

This volume will be extremely valuable for increasing reflective practice as well as increasing the skill of practitioners in tackling difficult ethical issues. In my opinion it should not only be in every hospital library, but it should also be a core text of any course in geriatric medicine.

**Jeremy R Playfer** MD FRCP
**Consultant Physician, Royal Liverpool University Hospital**
**President Elect, British Geriatrics Society**
*March 2004*

# Foreword

The rapid aging of the human population and the medical, ethical, and legal challenges associated with this phenomenon are matters of international significance in today's world. There are important differences in the ways in which the United Kingdom and the United States confront some of these challenges. Beyond distinctions in the unique jargon employed in each jurisdiction, there are certain differences in the details of common and statutory law relating to specific matters of mutual concern; regarding the confidentiality of patient information, for example, the UK is governed by the Data Protection Act of 1998 while medical entities in the US are scrambling to comply with recent regulations implementing the Health Insurance Portability and Accountability Act (HIPAA) of 1996. Perhaps the UK and US differ most in the geriatric medicine context in terms of their respective systems for financing the care of older persons, with the UK characterized by the national health service (supplemented by private pay) and the US relying on a combination of the newly revised federal government Medicare program, Medicaid for the indigent, private Medigap insurance policies, and out-of-pocket contributions.

Despite these differences, there are enormous similarities in the fundamental underlying cultural, ethical, and policy values and tensions affecting medical practitioners who treat the elderly in both the UK and US. Generic ethical issues with which both UK and American physicians regularly deal (such as respecting patient autonomy) take on special twists in the geriatric sphere, because of particular characteristics of older patients (for instance, a higher prevalence of severe mental impairment), their residential or family settings, and the distinguishing objectives of geriatric care (that is, ordinarily a focus on patient function and quality of life rather than simple longevity). In both jurisdictions, legal rules are essential to ethical analysis, because the law sets parameters or boundaries within which particular courses of ethical action may be contemplated. At the same time, despite the legal labyrinth increasingly imposed on contemporary medical practice on both sides of the Atlantic, it remains very difficult to effectively externally monitor and enforce ethical behavior in practice. Thus, as the contributors to this volume recognize, just as vital as abstract ethical principles and legal edits in shaping daily geriatric practice are the role of healthcare provider virtues and the values and preferences of older patients, their families, providers, and the community.

No book can make anyone become more ethical, but this volume will help ethical geriatric professionals deal appropriately with situations presenting inconsistent or even conflicting values, as those professionals search for the best, or the least worst, alternatives. There exists no mathematically precise formula for arriving at an ethically defensible course of behavior in any actual set of circumstances, but this volume provides the reader with a valuable initial framework for identifying, dissecting, and addressing major ethical concerns in geriatric practice.

In both the UK and US, geriatric ethics is very much an applied rather than an academic endeavor. In this volume, the parsing of numerous hypothetical cases should be an effective tool for promoting the sort of problem-based learning that has become popular in other parts of contemporary medical education.

Given the significant commonalities in underlying professional and social values, there is much that the UK and US geriatrics communities could teach to and learn from each other. In some respects, medical practitioners in the UK have been more honest and open about certain unpleasant ethical issues, most notably healthcare rationing (*see* Chapter 5), than their American counterparts, and the latter might profit from emulating the former in this respect. I hope that this fine book will not only immensely assist physicians, medical students, and other healthcare providers in the UK, but will also facilitate more communication and interaction between the UK and US geriatrics communities regarding the ethical questions and norms that they unavoidably share.

**Marshall B Kapp** JD MPH FCLM
**Arthur W Grayson Distinguished Professor of Law and Medicine**
**Southern Illinois University School of Law, USA**
*March 2004*

At the time this foreword was written, Marshall Kapp was Professor in the Departments of Community Health and Psychiatry and Director of the Office of Geriatric Medicine and Gerontology at Wright State University School of Medicine in Dayton, Ohio, as well as a member of the adjunct faculty at the University of Dayton School of Law.

# Preface

Since the publication of the first edition of this book in 1999 we have seen the introduction of the Human Rights Act 1998, which incorporates the European Convention of Human Rights into UK law, the production of new guidelines on cardiopulmonary resuscitation by the British Medical Association in 2002, the new draft bill on mental incapacity, the new guidelines on consent for treatment and the publication of the National Service Framework for Older People, with a commitment to abolish ageism in clinical practice. The updated chapters have included these changes in law, the new guidelines and the new standards set out in the National Service Framework for Older People. In addition, two important new chapters on confidentiality and on ethical issues and driving have been added.

However, the main aim of the book remains the same – it is intended to be a practical guide for junior medical staff, including specialist registrars. Other professionals who are involved with doctors in making difficult decisions will also find this text useful, as will medical students who now have to learn about medical ethics and their application in day-to-day management of patients, as part of the undergraduate curriculum.

# About the editor

**Gurcharan S Rai** is consultant physician at the Whittington Hospital, London and is a member of the British Geriatrics Society and of its Special Group on Medical Ethics, and a Fellow of the American Geriatrics Society. He has extensive experience in teaching and training of undergraduates and postgraduates and at the present time is Chair of the Training Committee and Regional Adviser for Geriatric Medicine in North Thames (East).

# List of contributors

**Iva Blackman**
Consultant Physician in Geriatric Medicine
Cirencester Hospital

**Ann Bowling**
Professor of Health Services Research
University College London

**Nick Coni**
Consultant Physician Emeritus
Addenbrooke's Hospital
Cambridge

**Olivier Gaillemin**
Specialist Registrar
South Manchester University Hospitals NHS Trust
Manchester

**Lalit Kalra**
Professor of Stroke Medicine
King's College Hospital
London

**Steven Luttrell**
Consultant Physician in Older People's Services
St Pancras Hospital
Medical Director, Camden Primary Care Trust

**Catherine McAdam**
Specialist Registrar, Care of Older People
Whittington Hospital
London

**Desmond O'Neill**
Associate Professor
Department of Gerontology, Trinity Centre for Health Services
Adelaide and Meath Hospital
Dublin

**Kamilla K Porter**
GP Registrar
Holland Park, London

**Donald Portsmouth**
Honorary Senior Clinical Lecturer
Centre for Biomedical Ethics
University of Birmingham

**Rachel Powis**
Specialist Registrar
Royal Hampshire County Hospital
Winchester

**Gurdeep S Rai**
Postgraduate Law Student

**David Robinson**
Associate Professor
Department of Gerontology, Trinity Centre for Health Sciences
Adelaide and Meath Hospital
Dublin

**Kevin Stewart**
Consultant Geriatrician
Royal Hampshire County Hospital
Winchester

**David Sulch**
Consultant Physician
Queen Elizabeth Hospital
London

**Martin J Vernon**
Consultant Physician in Elderly Medicine
Wythenshawe Hospital
Manchester

# CHAPTER 1

# Principles of medical ethics

## Kamilla K Porter and Gurcharan S Rai

Medical knowledge and technology have advanced at a spectacular rate. This voyage of discovery has led to a wealth of ethical issues unimaginable to the original followers of the Hippocratic oath. Steeped in the history of philosophy and religion, the development of medical ethics has been an attempt to unravel and resolve the moral complexities and dilemmas that have faced doctors through the ages. Several tenets of medical ethics have stood the test of time and are embraced by modern-day ethical guidelines – for example, *primum non nocere* (first do no harm). Other concepts, such as the notion of communal responsibility and justice, have arisen in the complex modern medical era. What the twenty-first century medical practitioner requires is a comprehensive framework to help in the identification of and critical reflection on ethical problems.

There are four widely accepted general principles of medical ethics which go towards such a framework, namely *autonomy, justice, beneficence* and *nonmaleficence*. This 'four cluster' model of moral principles central to biomedical ethics was pioneered by the ethicists Beauchamp and Childress.[1] This approach has met with some criticism as being too simplistic, but of great appeal is that these prima facie principles offer flexibility, represent a neutral frame of reference applicable to patients from different cultures and religions and are independent of political doctrines.[2] There has been a proliferation of ethical guidelines from different medical professional bodies such as the General Medical Council (GMC) and medical defence organisations with regard to clinical practice as well as local and national ethical codes with regard to research. In addition, the 1998 Human Rights Act has had an impact on ethical decisions in the setting of healthcare. For example, Article 2 (right to life), Article 3 (right to freedom from inhuman and degrading treatment) and Article 14 (right to be free from discriminatory practices such as ageism) will affect policies relating to resuscitation orders, aspects of palliative care practice and the level of care in nursing homes.[3]

The profile of patient autonomy has also been raised further as the media and the Internet have provided the public with greater access to information on medicine and health. The 'four-principle' approach discussed in this introductory chapter does not serve as a manual with precise instructions, but rather it provides a framework with which to analyse and critically reflect upon ethical problems and guidelines. A useful way of thinking about the four-principle model is to consider each principle as one of the four nucleotides that constitute 'moral DNA', capable in combination or on their own of clarifying and justifying the general norms that underlie healthcare ethics.[4]

# Autonomy

Autonomy is about respecting patients' wishes and facilitating and encouraging their input into the medical decision-making process. The issue of informed consent and refusal lies at the heart of this principle. To respect a patient's autonomy is to give that individual a greater balance of power in the doctor–patient relationship. It entails explaining not only what is wrong with that person, but also the options and implications of any proposed investigation and treatment and the associated risks and benefits. The practitioner needs to provide the patient with as much information as he or she both wishes for and requires in order to make a decision.

Such information needs to be delivered in a clear and concise manner. A balance must be struck between confusing the individual with medical jargon and adopting an overly simplified approach that fails to include important details. The art of pitching the consultation at the right level is by no means straightforward, but where possible by ensuring that the patient understands his or her particular medical problem and management options the doctor should avoid the pitfall of using his or her own personal value system to judge what is best for the patient.

The issue of autonomy is all the more poignant among the elderly population in a society where older people can lose respect and personal choice. With its emphasis on patient-centred care and rooting out age discrimination, the National Service Framework for Older People is promoting greater autonomy among the elderly, highlighting 'the need to view service users as active participants in, rather than subjects of, the care-providing process'.[5]

The application of the principle of autonomy can be seen in the following case of an 80-year-old diabetic woman who was admitted to hospital with cardiac failure following a myocardial infarction. Her mental faculties were fully intact and she was making a steady recovery when her foot became ischaemic. Conservative management was instigated, but the foot could not be salvaged. The vascular surgeons explained on several occasions that in order to curtail the ascending ischaemia and to prevent potentially life-threatening infection, she needed a below-knee amputation. She was informed of her considerable anaesthetic risk, as well as the likelihood of remaining in hospital for several weeks after surgery and then needing a substantial care package. The patient requested time to talk to her family, and after further discussion with both the physicians and surgeons she declined surgery. Over the ensuing days her leg became gangrenous and she died from overwhelming sepsis. The case sparked differing viewpoints among the medical staff, some of whom felt that with the option of local anaesthetic block instead of a general anaesthetic, it was worth risking surgery to prevent this hitherto active and vibrant individual dying from sepsis. Others felt that with dedicated nursing care and good pain control, the patient's refusal to go ahead with surgery was preferable to a long and complicated recovery period and loss of her independent lifestyle.

This case scenario illustrates how, when management options are no longer clear-cut, the patient can play a pivotal role in guiding the doctor through an ethical maze. The principle of autonomy, although a noble ideal, is not without its limitations. Patients may be unable to contribute fully to discussions about their care for a variety of reasons – for example, in an emergency situation when swift intervention is needed, or when there are communication difficulties which could be due to cultural and language barriers or practical problems such as impairment after a stroke. Furthermore, some patients may reject opportunities to exercise their autonomy and request that the doctor acts on their behalf, as is evident in the statement 'whatever you think best, doctor'. Under such circumstances the doctor has to decide what course of action would be most appropriate for the patient, but only after they have given that patient the option of sharing in the decision-making process.

Doctors themselves may feel threatened and challenged by involving patients in making decisions about treatment – for example, due to time constraints in a busy clinic or surgery and a lack of appropriate information to support patients' decisions. Some doctors may feel uncomfortable and lack the skills to negotiate a decision with the patient.[6] This is an area of ongoing research and one which has implications for medical training. It has been argued that failing to accommodate patients' needs and preferences will ultimately diminish doctors' standing.[7]

Respecting autonomy becomes more complicated in cases of mental incompetence. Deciding how to treat the elderly woman with the ischaemic foot would have been more difficult if she had also been suffering from dementia. In such situations the doctor is obliged to look beyond the individual in the sick bed and to consider the patient in the context of her home and family – in other words, taking into account quality-of-life issues. Other health professionals, family members and carers can provide invaluable information. The patient may have made her wishes clear to relatives before her mental deterioration, or in the form of a living will or advance directive. The ethical reverberations of mental incompetence and the issues of living wills, advance directives and quality-of-life measurements are examined in detail in later chapters.

# Justice

In the context of healthcare, justice implies an impartial and fair approach to treatment and the distribution of resources. Doctors discriminate unfairly if they allow their prejudices to directly influence their professional work. Established ethical and human rights codes condemn any form of discrimination on the grounds of age, race, sex, religion or sexual orientation. Can an individual forfeit their entitlement to medical care as a result of their lifestyle or antisocial behaviour directly leading to ill health? Examples would include patients with peripheral vascular disease who continue to smoke, intravenous drug users who have contracted hepatitis or HIV, or people with obesity-related problems who fail to adhere to diet and exercise regimes. If, despite appropriate advice and information about the dangers of high-risk activities such as smoking, a patient continues to take that risk, accepting their decision is effectively taking into account that patient's autonomy. At the same time, encouraging the patient to take responsibility for their medical problems is also to respect their autonomy.

However, as the cost of healthcare continues to spiral, the issue of social justice and the needs of other health service users cannot be overlooked. Would it be fair to withhold treatment for those who engage in voluntary risk taking at the expense of their health? There are no easy answers to this question, and it is difficult to attribute an individual's ill health solely to their personal actions, as genetic, environmental and social factors can also play a role. Furthermore, some risk taking can result in less rather than more healthcare costs, as such individuals may die earlier and more quickly than those who engage in a less risky lifestyle.[8]

A caring society demands that limited resources are allocated in a just manner. The *Oxford Dictionary of Philosophy* defines distributive justice as 'the link between a distributive system and the maximisation of well-being'. Difficulties arise because of the inevitable scarcity of resources and subsequent conflicts between competing speciality groups. Increasingly, health professionals and governments are confronted with legitimate competing concerns and are having to acknowledge the prioritisation of patient needs. When a potential treatment is wanted for a patient, the final decision may be that due to the overwhelming need of others, the purchasing of this expensive treatment cannot be justified. Examples of such outcomes include the withdrawal by some health authorities of infertility treatment, and the prescription of certain drugs on the NHS such as interferon for multiple sclerosis not being permitted by some health authorities. Partly in response to the perceived unfairness of such decisions, numerous national and local clinical guidelines have emerged in recent years. These do not necessarily take the sting out of the tail when an individual is denied his or her wishes, and a difficult balance has to be struck between personal autonomy and the benefit to society at large.

In an era of increasing healthcare costs, an ageing population and development of more sophisticated treatments and procedures, the issue of healthcare rationing cannot be avoided. Central to this issue are questions of what we mean by human dignity and what level of basic care can still be deemed humane. Setting and defining the limits of an acceptable level of minimum medical care is a dynamic process that requires input from medical professionals, politicians, health managers and the general public. It has been argued that at the very least the aim of basic healthcare is to prevent premature death, to enable an individual to function as a productive member of society and, when that is no longer possible, to alleviate distressing symptoms for the remaining duration of that individual's life and as he or she approaches death.[9]

# Beneficence and non-maleficence

The doctor should act to promote the welfare of his or her patient and to do good (beneficence). An action that is taken to benefit the patient may entail risks, so at the same time we have to consider the principle of non-maleficence (to avoid doing harm). In essence we are looking at a cost : benefit ratio, and it is of critical importance that it is patient centred. Acting in the best interests of the patient is a stance that also incorporates respecting autonomy, and conflicts can arise between these principles. Consider the patient who requests an investigation or treatment which the doctor finds to be unwarranted clinically – for example, a lumbar spine X-ray for an episode of mild lower back pain. The doctor's refusal could be seen as paternalistic, and the patient may feel aggrieved, but the doctor has to weigh up the risks and merits of the intervention requested against the patient's wishes and the preservation of a good doctor–patient relationship.

Sometimes the risk of harm to others in the population needs to be taken into account, and the principle of non-maleficence may outweigh the patient's autonomy. An example would be the detention in hospital of a patient who has pulmonary tuberculosis and has repeatedly failed to take their medication regularly in the community. Such drastic action has been deemed ethical on the grounds of the infective risk that the patient poses to the public, and the possibility that he could develop multi-drug resistance and become more unwell through his haphazard use of medication.

Deciding what is beneficial overall to the patient and what constitutes harm can be fraught with difficulty, particularly with regard to end-of-life decisions such as withholding or withdrawing treatment and the much debated issue of euthanasia and physician-assisted suicide. The notion of saving life underpins medical training. However, nowadays there is also a greater emphasis on examining the quality of life and the concept of dignified death. In the UK, where euthanasia is illegal, doctors follow the doctrine of double effect, under which it is permissible to administer medication to alleviate distressing symptoms of terminal illness even though the patient may die sooner as a result, but the doctor has to prove that the objective is to relieve suffering, not to shorten life. The fear is that if doctors actively assisted patients in ending their lives, the door would be opened to a slippery slope towards involuntary euthanasia where the old or frail might be put under pressure by relatives or be made to feel like an unwanted burden to their families and society. Some argue that there is a very thin line between respecting a terminally ill patient's refusal of life-sustaining treatment and yet turning down their request for assistance in directly ending their life in order to avoid more suffering.[10] These topics will be explored further in later chapters.

# Conclusion

Healthcare professionals require an ethical basis for their day-to-day work. The four general principles outlined above, although they have been described separately, are interlinked and can be employed on their own or in combination. This model has its limitations and does not necessarily provide us with obvious answers, but it serves as a useful framework for the identification and analysis of ethical problems.

From doing something seemingly straightforward such as performing a blood test to completing do-not-resuscitate orders, doctors are making ethical decisions – taking into account the patient's wishes (respecting his or her *autonomy*), weighing up the benefits against the possible harm of any medical action (*beneficence* and *non-maleficence*) and taking into consideration whether that action and its cost are fair overall (exercising *justice*).

The onus of such decision making no longer rests with the doctor alone. The media, the Internet and patient groups and advocates are providing the public with information about medicine and health on an unprecedented scale. This trend, together with the passing of the Human Rights Act, has brought the issue of patient autonomy to even greater prominence. Developments in biotechnology and research pose many moral questions, and with increasing medical specialisation, ethical decision making requires the engagement not only of the patient and the healthcare professional but also of society at large.

# References

1   Beauchamp TL and Childress JF (1979) *Principles of Biomedical Ethics* (1e). Oxford University Press, New York.

2   Gillon R (1994) Medical ethics: four principles plus attention to scope. *BMJ.* **309**: 184–8.

3  Hewson B (2000) Why the Human Rights Act matters to doctors. *BMJ.* **321**: 780–1.

4  Gillon R (2003) Ethics needs principles – four can encompass the rest – and respect for autonomy should be 'first among equals'. *J Med Ethics.* **29**: 307–12.

5  www.doh.gov.uk/nsf/olderpeople.htm

6  Say RE and Thomson R (2003) The importance of patient preferences in treatment decisions – challenges for doctors. *BMJ.* **327**: 542–5.

7  Coulter A (2002) Patients' views of the good doctor. *BMJ.* **325**: 668–9.

8  Beauchamp TL and Childress JF (2001) *Principles of Biomedical Ethics* (5e). Oxford University Press, New York.

9  Garrett TM, Baillie HW and Garret RM (1993) *Health Care: ethics, principles and problems* (3e). Prentice-Hall, Inc., New Jersey.

10  Doyal L and Doyal L (2001) Why active euthanasia and physician-assisted suicide should be legalised. *BMJ.* **323**: 1079–80.

## Further reading and useful websites

- Beauchamp TL and Childress JF (2001) *Principles of Biomedical Ethics* (5e). Oxford University Press, New York.

- Garrett TM, Ballie HW and Garrett RM (2001) *Health Care: ethics, principles and problems.* Prentice-Hall, Inc.

- Campbell AV, Charlesworth M, Gillett G and Jones G (2001) *Medical Ethics.* Oxford University Press, Oxford.

- UK Clinical Ethics Network www.ethics-network.org.uk

- Journal of Medical Ethics www.jmedethics.com

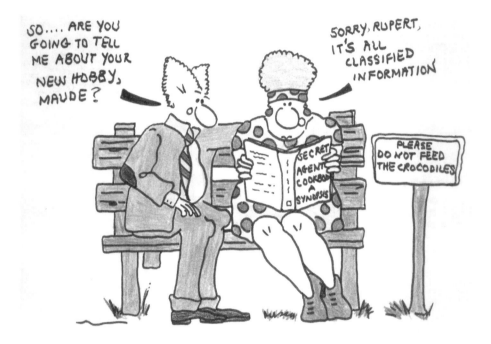

# CHAPTER 2

# Confidentiality

## *Catherine McAdam and Gurcharan S Rai*

Confidentiality is one of the basic premises of medical practice and was enshrined in the Hippocratic oath:

> Whatever, in connection with my professional practice or not in connection with it, I see or hear, in the life of men, which ought not to be spoken of abroad, I will not divulge, as reckoning that all such should be kept secret.

This concept is now expressed in the professional codes of practice of healthcare professionals around the world. In the UK it is laid out in the General Medical Council's *Duties of a Doctor*. It states that doctors have a duty to respect the privacy of patients and to protect the information divulged to them in confidence. Any information obtained in a professional capacity is subject to this. Consent should always be obtained before sharing this information with others, unless there are exceptional circumstances. Confidentiality is fundamental to a doctor–patient relationship based on trust, but doctors also have a duty of care to the community at large. This, coupled with the nature of information shared between doctors and their patients, can lead to conflicts of interest. When these occur and the question of breaching confidentiality arises, there must be clear ethical justification for doing so.

In addition, it is worth noting that the Human Rights Act 1998 includes a right to freedom of expression under Article 10, and this also prevents healthcare staff from disclosing information that has been given to them in confidence.

## The importance of confidentiality

The need for confidentiality is based on two principles:

1  the patient's right to privacy and autonomy
2  the preservation of a doctor–patient relationship that is based on mutual trust.

We choose carefully the information that we share with others. This information helps us to shape our identity – how we view ourselves, how we want others to see us and, to an extent, how they actually perceive us. Patients divulge sensitive information to their doctors about their physical, emotional, social and sexual health that they may not share with anyone else. The assumption of confidentiality means that they can do this without fear of embarrassment or disapproval. Without an implicit understanding that information will be kept private, patients may feel unable to talk to their doctor openly and frankly. This impediment to good communication could make the already challenging task of appropriate investigation and therapy even more difficult. The fears of HIV and AIDS patients in the 1980s and 1990s illustrated the wide-ranging consequences of compromising confidentiality. There are implications for an individual's personal relationships, work and finance, as well as the possibility of discrimination.

In reality, the public's perception of what confidentiality means and the practice of modern medicine may differ significantly. This is in part because of the increasing numbers of people involved in providing medical care. It is particularly true when caring for the elderly, where those involved can range from nursing staff and physiotherapists to carers and day-hospital receptionists. It is unlikely that patients are aware of the extent to which personal information is disseminated. There has also been an expansion in those who are not directly involved in patient care but who are involved in research and administration. Computerised records, more widespread technical support services and the expansion of databases can also be seen to threaten our traditional notion of confidentiality.

Perhaps more pertinent for the majority of patients is how we deal with sensitive information on a busy ward or in a local general practice. Often life-changing discussions, such as the breaking of bad news, are conducted with just a curtain separating the patient from the outside world. Similarly, patients are openly discussed on a ward within hearing distance of other patients and relatives. Indiscretion is arguably the commonest form of breach of confidentiality. This may, for example, take the form of leaving information unguarded on a computer screen or talking about patients to a colleague in a hospital canteen. Lapses can also occur when we are caring for older people who are very frail or with whom we find it difficult to communicate (e.g. due to deafness or dysarthria). We may find it simpler to talk to their next of kin. More detailed information is sometimes revealed to relatives and carers than to patients, without having ensured their consent.

# Sharing information with the patient's consent

Consent must be obtained before disclosing information to another party, unless lack of consent is dictated by exceptional circumstances. It is good practice to document this consent. Depending on the nature of the disclosure, this can be done formally with the patient's written consent or as a record that verbal consent has been given. To give their consent, the patient should understand the nature and effects of the disclosure and have the capacity to make the decision.

It is essential that information is shared between health professionals in order to provide good healthcare. Clearly it is not always necessary to obtain explicit consent for this, provided that the patient has agreed to treatment or investigation. For instance, if a patient agrees to a specialist referral from their general practitioner (GP), then it is implied that they are happy for the GP to pass on details to the specialist. Patients expect health professionals to communicate in their best interests, and poor communication is a common source of frustration. However, difficulties can arise when patients and their doctors differ in their understanding of what information needs to be communicated and to whom. Only information that is relevant and required for optimum care should be disclosed, and it is the doctor's duty to ensure that the patient understands what information will be given.

If information is to be shared with others who are not involved in the healthcare of a patient, such as an employer, then the patient's consent must be obtained. This should be done in writing prior to disclosure, and should be limited to relevant information. It is the doctor's responsibility to ensure that the patient is aware of any adverse effects such disclosures may have.

---

**Case 1**
Mrs J is an active 87-year-old. She is admitted as an emergency with dehydration due to vomiting. An endoscopy reveals a gastric malignancy that is inoperable. On being told of the diagnosis, Mrs J is adamant that she does not want her family to be made aware of it. She says that she does not want her family treating her 'like an invalid', and she wants to 'enjoy what is left of her life'. She has a large, caring extended family who until this point have been fully informed of events, and who now want to know what is wrong with Mrs J.

**Comment**
Mrs J's wishes should be respected. It may be helpful to discuss with her the impact of the decision. She may find it difficult to carry the burden of illness

alone and find it hard to plan the rest of her time without the assistance of her family. At some stage in the course of her illness it is likely that they will discover the diagnosis and will be hurt that they did not know about it sooner. Most importantly, dialogue should be kept open with Mrs J, as her views may change over time.

# Sharing information without consent

It is not always possible to obtain consent to divulge personal information. This can occur in an emergency situation where it is not practicable to do so, or when patients decide to withhold consent or do not have the capacity to give it. In the UK, the principle of confidentiality is not considered absolute. The General Medical Council offers guidance on situations when doctors may be justified in or required to disclose information that has been imparted to them in confidence. These can be summarised as follows:

1   when it is in the best interests of the patient
2   when it is in the public interest
3   when it is required by statute or law
4   for the purposes of medical research and education, or public health.

In cases where it has not been possible to obtain consent, the patient should be informed of the decision to disclose information at the earliest opportunity. Breaching confidentiality, even when justifiable, remains an infringement of the patient's rights, and doctors should be prepared to defend these decisions. It may be advisable to discuss the matter with a colleague or a professional body before arriving at such a decision.

# In the patient's or public's best interests

It is sometimes necessary to divulge information in the best interests of a patient or the public, or when required by statute (e.g. cases of notifiable disease), without consent. Difficulties most often arise when a patient will not give consent but a doctor feels obliged to reveal information. In such a situation the potential benefits of making a disclosure need to be carefully weighed against the harm caused to the patient and the loss of faith in the medical profession for that patient and for others. Attempts should always be made to persuade the patient to share information voluntarily or to give their consent to this. It might be helpful to ask the patient hypothetically what they would do if they were in the doctor's position. A commonly encountered example is a patient with epilepsy, who is considered unfit to drive because of the condition, but continues to do so against medical advice and will not inform the driving authorities. If a doctor is unable to persuade him or her to stop driving, then telling the medical adviser of the Driver and Vehicle Licensing Agency (DVLA) can be justified, and the patient should be made aware of this.

---

### Case 2

Ms C is diagnosed as having a hereditary condition. As the family doctor you also look after her sister, who is undergoing IVF treatment in the hope of conceiving a child. The risk to Ms C's sister of developing this debilitating and fatal illness is significant. Ms C refuses to tell her family of her condition, although she is aware of the implications for her sister and any children she may have.

### Comment

You must balance the autonomy of Ms C against that of her sister. Disclosing information to the sister will be seen as a breach of trust by Ms C, and will damage your relationship. However, there is potential for harm to the sister in terms of her own health and the risk of conceiving an affected child. There are also consequences for the child and for the society which will share the burden. Ultimately these value judgements can only be made by the mother, but she is entitled to the information to enable her to do this. This warrants disclosing the information to the sister. If Ms C cannot be convinced of this, then she should be made aware of your intentions to tell her sister.

---

Decisions where there is conflict between the rights of known individuals and of others are most challenging when the degree and probability of harm are hard to quantify. A doctor's duty to the public may prevail if a disclosure may assist in the prevention, detection or prosecution of serious crime. If there is a risk of death or serious harm then the doctor is required to disclose information. Again, only relevant information should be shared and it should not be used for other purposes.

---

### Case 3

Mr W is a 75-year-old who has been admitted with a chest infection. He is thin and unkempt and has a number of bruises on his arms and chest. He lives with his son and relies on him for assistance with personal care and to do the shopping and cooking. Nursing staff raise the possibility of abuse. Mr W will not discuss the matter and says that he wants to go home to his son.

**Comment**
There are no specific laws in the UK to protect the elderly from abuse. Mr W is dependent on a close family member who may be guilty of neglect or abuse. However, he remains a competent adult capable of making his own decisions. If you feel that Mr W is at risk of serious harm, alerting the police can be justified. If this is not the case, then it should not be discussed with those who are not immediately involved in his care or with his son. It may be prudent to suggest supportive measures for the patient. The introduction of a care package may help to ease the burden of care for his son, and will ensure a point of contact with external services should Mr W need further assistance.

# Legal process

In a court of law a judge can order the disclosure of information. A doctor can object if he or she believes the information to be irrelevant, but the decision falls to the judge. Information should not be given to either lawyers or police without consent. The only exception to this is where failure to disclose information would put people at risk of serious harm. Information must also be disclosed if there is a statutory obligation to do so – for example, in the notification of certain infectious diseases or in cases of substance misuse.

The Data Protection Act 1998 and Access to Health Records Act 1990 gives health professionals the right not to disclose information if they believe that disclosure is likely to cause serious harm to the physical or mental health of the patient or any other person.

# Medical research, education and public health

It is widely accepted that information obtained in clinical practice is used for other purposes, including medical research and education, audit, epidemiology and health planning. These do not directly benefit the patient, but are of use to society as a whole. While sharing much of this kind of information poses little threat to the patient, it has still been imparted in confidence, and the use and protection of this data has been controversial. In broad terms, information should only be given to those who are also bound by a duty of confidentiality, consent should be sought to share information, and data should be anonymous if this will suffice.

---

**Case 4**

Mrs B's family comes to visit her in hospital. They are incensed to find a medical student reading their mother's notes at the nurse's desk.

**Comment**

The value of confidentiality needs to be impressed upon medical students and other trainee health professionals from an early stage of their training. Most patients recognise the importance of medical education and are keen to assist in it. It can be argued that the medical student in this case should have obtained consent to read the notes, as they would have done before taking a history from the patient or carrying out a physical examination.

---

More and more data are being stored on information technology systems. This has been accompanied by increasing public concern about what information is stored and how it can be accessed. The Data Protection Act 1998 safeguards patient information that is held on computer. In addition, the NHS Information Authority is producing guidelines on the management of information. It is also considering ways to promote public awareness of how such data are used to improve standards of care.

In medical research, consent should be sought to use information if it is practicable to do so. Data should be made anonymous where possible. If information is identifiable and it is not practicable to obtain consent, then the local ethics and research committee should be consulted on the best way to proceed.

# Release of information after death

---

**Case 5**

The nephew of an 89-year-old Greek patient, who had attended an outpatient department for investigations and management of diabetes and abnormal liver function tests a year earlier, makes an appointment to see the consultant. At the meeting he informs the consultant that his aunt died six months ago and before her death her brother made her sign a will while she was ill in hospital. According to the will his aunt has left all of her estate to her brother. However, the nephew suspects that this will does not represent the true wishes of his aunt, for it is written in English and she could not speak or write English. He asks for copies of medical records which state that his aunt could not communicate in English and that at each outpatient visit an interpreter was required.

**Comment**

While it would be only natural to sympathise with the nephew, it would be wrong to go along with his request. Under the Access to Health Records Act 1990, only a deceased person's representative can access such information. There is a general misconception that a deceased person's next of kin is the personal representative. This is not necessarily the case. If a will is made, then it is the executor of the will who is the lawful personal representative. If no will is made and the deceased died intestate, it is at this stage that the closest 'next of kin' can apply, through a solicitor, for a Letter of Administration to handle the deceased's affairs. In this case it is the deceased person's brother who has a statutory right to access to health information.

In most cases an application for access to medical records is made in relation to an insurance claim. No information (and this includes results of investigations) can be revealed to a third party which the patient gave in the past on the understanding that it would be kept confidential. Importantly, doctors should not disclose any information if the patient has requested non-disclosure and this is documented in the medical records.

# Access to medical reports

Medical reports commonly prepared by practitioners for employment and insurance purposes are based on confidential information provided by an individual to the doctor. Under the Access to Medical Reports Act 1988, the patient has a right to inspect or be supplied with a copy of medical reports. However, a report prepared by an independent practitioner who has not treated the person and who has never been involved in his or her care is not covered by the Medical Reports Act 1988 or the Data Protection Act 1998.

**Key points**

- Doctors have a duty to keep any information that is learned in a professional capacity confidential.
- Disclosures should only be made with a patient's consent, except in exceptional circumstances.
- In addition to the Access to Health Records Act 1990, the Human Rights Act 1998 (the right to freedom) confirms a responsibility to prevent disclosure of information that has been imparted in confidence.
- Only information that is relevant for the provision of good healthcare should be disclosed. Patients should be made aware of what information has been divulged.

- Careful consideration must be given to breaking the confidence of a patient. Doctors must be able to justify these breaches.
- Information to be used in education, research or for public health interests should be anonymous where possible.
- The health records of a deceased person must be treated as confidential records, and only Executor of the Will, who is the lawful personal representative, has a statutory right to access the health records.

# Further reading

- General Medical Council (2000) *Protecting Patients, Guiding Doctors. Confidentiality: protecting and providing information*. General Medical Council, London.

- Siegler M (1982) Confidentiality in medicine – a decrepit concept. *NEJM*. **307**: 1518–21.

- Beauchamp TL and Childress JF (1994) Professional–patient relationships. In: *Principles of Biomedical Ethics* (4e). Oxford University Press, New York.

- British Medical Association's Ethics, Science and Information Division (1993) Confidentiality and medical records. In: *Medical Ethics Today. Its practice and philosophy*. British Medical Association, London.

- Mason JK, McCall Smith RA and Laurie GT (2002) Medical confidentiality. In: G Laurie (ed.) *Law and Medical Ethics* (6e). Butterworths, London.

- NHS Information Authority (2003) *Protecting Patient Confidentiality*; www.nhsia.nhs.uk/confidentiality.

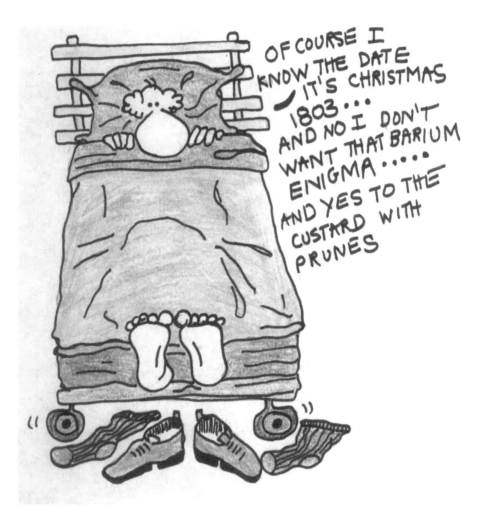

# CHAPTER 3

# Informed consent

*Martin J Vernon*

## Introduction

The last decade has seen positive and sustained movement towards person-centred care for older people.[1,2] Patient choice is a central value and fundamental to good medical practice.[3] Few would contemplate forcing treatment on an individual against their wishes or without first seeking their views. Consent pervades all aspects of clinical work, and yet it often remains nothing more than a mundane procedure which begins and ends with the signing of a consent form. In many situations the consent process passes off without difficulty, sometimes even unnoticed by the parties concerned. However, when the process breaks down, health workers are often left wondering how best to proceed. In these circumstances an understanding of the underlying professional, moral and legal issues can help to resolve the dilemmas which ensue.

Healthcare for older people is particularly fraught with problems concerning consent. Physical and mental impairments may hinder the normal dialogue which occurs between carer and patient, thereby obstructing the usual consent process. At worst this leads to a complete failure of the process, either because the patient is unable or unwilling to *provide* consent, or because the carer is unable or unwilling to *seek* consent. The following familiar case examples illustrate these problems.

---

**Case 1**  a patient unable to provide consent

Dr Smith wishes to obtain a sample of blood from her patient, Harry, who suffers from dementia and is profoundly confused. He spends much of his day staring out of a window and rarely talks. The doctor tries to explain her intentions to Harry, but he cries out loudly and pulls away when she lifts his arm and tries to insert the needle.

---

---

**Case 2** a patient unwilling to provide consent

Dr Smith wishes to obtain a sample of blood from her patient, Freda, who is awaiting surgery for a fractured neck of femur. The doctor tries to explain her intentions, but Freda shrugs and says that at her time of life she does not want to be 'pulled about' and is much happier being left alone, 'whatever the consequences'.

---

**Case 3** a carer unable to seek consent

Dr Smith wishes to obtain a sample of blood from her patient, Hilda, who has severely impaired hearing. The doctor tries to explain her intentions to Hilda, who smiles but does not otherwise respond. Dr Smith is left feeling uncertain as to how much has been understood.

---

**Case 4** a carer unwilling to seek consent

Dr Smith wishes to obtain a sample of blood from her patient, Jack, who has suffered a stroke and has expressive dysphasia. The doctor tries to explain her intentions to Jack, who attempts to respond but struggles to get the words out. Dr Smith listens to him struggling for a few minutes, but is in a hurry and decides to proceed before Jack has finished trying to express himself. He becomes tearful during the procedure, and the doctor later worries about the correctness of her actions.

---

By presenting a structured approach to the consent process, this chapter seeks to provide assistance in resolving dilemmas which are commonly encountered in delivering healthcare to older people. While it is tempting to resort to legal frameworks when deciding right from wrong, there are many situations where the law is unhelpful or even silent. A more pragmatic approach is first to consider the *moral* basis of the consent process, and to work from first principles towards a solution which is *consistent* with the law, rather than dictated by it.

# The basis of consent

## Professional duties

It is helpful to look at the values which underlie the duties of health professionals. The various strands of professional practice on which the notion of consent is based are readily discernible in a variety of professional mandates. For example, in the Hippocratic oath attention is drawn to the importance of acting only for a patient's benefit, and avoiding doing them harm:

> I will prescribe regimen for the good of my patients according to my ability and judgement and never do harm to anyone. ... In every house where I come I will enter only for the good of my patients, keeping myself far from all intentional ill-doing.[4]

More recently, the General Medical Council, in setting out the duties of a doctor, has focused on the importance of consent in maintaining trust:

> Patients must be able to trust doctors with their lives and well-being. ... In particular, as a doctor you must:

> - treat every patient politely and considerately
> - listen to patients and respect their views
> - give patients information in a way they can understand
> - respect the rights of patients to be fully involved in decisions about their care
> - make sure that your personal beliefs do not prejudice your patients' care.[3]

## The moral basis of consent

Although specifically directed towards doctors, intuitively these declarations are more generally applicable. On closer inspection, three common themes emerge:

- avoidance of doing intentional harm
- promotion of benefit and well-being
- respect for the wishes and desires of the individual.

Each of these relates to a particular moral principle, and it is helpful to briefly consider each of them in turn.

### Non-maleficence

This principle creates an obligation not to do intentional harm to others, and there are a number of ways of achieving this. Most obviously we should try not to do things which cause harm, but we may also be obliged to stop or prevent processes which are causing harm to an individual. It is helpful to decide what we mean by *harm* in this situation. Although we ordinarily think of harm as meaning physical or psychological injury, there are other ways in which the interests of an individual may be damaged.

Returning to Dr Smith and her blood samples, we might conclude that Harry has been physically harmed when he cries out on being touched, but Jack's tearfulness also suggests harm, despite his showing no resistance to the procedure. This may be more than the pain of having blood taken, and may equally well relate to his thwarted attempts to express a view. In Freda's case, the patient has expressed clearly that she does not want a blood test and that she is best left alone. Ignoring her wishes would both undermine her interests in being left alone and damage the trust that she maintains with her carers. Such action may thus harm the integrity of future decision making.

### Beneficence

This principle requires us to act so as to contribute to the welfare of individuals, and it is closely allied to non-maleficence. We might choose to do this by actively providing benefit for a person, or by not restricting *opportunities* for benefit. Alternatively, we may choose to balance the benefits and drawbacks of a situation in order to arrive at the best outcome.

Dr Smith's cases provide some illustration of this principle. Her intention in obtaining the blood samples is presumably to derive information which will contribute to the welfare of her patients. By having open discussions with the patients she has sought to avoid restricting their opportunities. If the patient has expressed a view, at least it can be taken into account. By balancing the benefits and drawbacks for her patient, the doctor may be better placed to arrive at a decision on how to proceed. Such a calculation would depend on factors such as the magnitude of benefit to be derived from doing the test, and the amount of harm done by overriding any objections that the patient might have.

### Respect for autonomy

Respect for the wishes of an individual is perhaps at the root of morally robust consent. The concept of autonomy, although difficult to grasp, comprises elements of *freedom from interference* and *capacity for action*. In deciding whether to be influenced by an individual's views, it is useful to consider whether they are or can be autonomous. One view is that someone is autonomous if they:

- have plans free from interference by others
- have thought about these plans critically
- are free to carry out their plans.

Thinking about Dr Smith's patients, it could be argued that Harry's dementia prevents him from being autonomous. He does not appear to have the mental capacity to think about any plans. If he does have plans, his impairment is likely to constrain him in their execution. It could be argued that overriding his refusal does not conflict with the principle of respect for autonomy, since he is not autonomous. Freda, on the other hand, clearly wants to be left alone, 'whatever the consequences', indicating that she has at least considered that there may be consequences to her refusing the test. Adherents to the principle of respect for autonomy would be unable to justify overriding her refusal, unless other grounds for questioning her autonomy could be found.

Where there is sufficient evidence that an individual is autonomous, it is difficult to justify proceeding in the face of a clear refusal. However, where the evidence to establish autonomy is lacking, decisions about an individual's autonomy can be difficult. In this situation it is useful to consider instead the notion of an *autonomous choice*.[5] What matters here is whether the individual has *actually* made a free decision about their care, rather than whether they are capable of being autonomous. Dr Smith and her patients provide a useful illustration of this. Although Harry's dementia deprives him of autonomous status, he has nevertheless clearly indicated that he does not want a needle stuck in his arm. Whatever the reason for this response, it is a powerful demonstration that, despite his dementia, he can still state a preference to be left alone.

# Problems with respect for autonomy

Is there an over-reliance on the principle of respect for autonomy? While a patient retains autonomy we should respect their choices, whatever the outcome and so long as others are not harmed as a consequence. When autonomy is absent, the patient's views are no longer central to decision making. In a way this lets health workers off the moral hook. They need no longer worry about a patient who is choosing 'unwisely', because that choice does not demand respect. Instead, the views of others decide what should happen. Strict adherence to the principle of respect for autonomy could paradoxically lead to higher levels of paternalism if health workers are reluctant to grant their patients autonomous status.

The problem arises from the view that autonomy is either present or absent. The solution lies with willingness to permit 'partial autonomy' and to treat patients as people. The right to determine what should happen to oneself could therefore be granted on either ability to choose or preservation of self (personhood).

# Partial autonomy

Even in a 'free' society there are rules which restrict action and choice, so that no adult is completely autonomous. It is simply unrealistic to require a patient to have full autonomy before respecting their choices. However, surely a patient who is able to order and choose between their various desires (e.g. to eat, mobilise, or be free from pain) is deserving of respect? Arguably only a patient who exhibits no such ability should be excluded from the consent process.

# Personhood

Loss of this characteristic may indeed justify excluding the patient from a decision about their healthcare. However, many individuals without full autonomy will continue to be recognised as persons. The presence of actions that display purpose, awareness and intent together with a recognition of 'self' by external observers should prompt respect for preservation of personhood. Despite his dementia, Harry still presents himself as a person to his carers. Arguably the doctor should respect his choice because he remains a person despite partial or even absent autonomy.

# The anatomy of consent

Consent in clinical practice may assume a variety of guises, from an explicit, fully informed dialogue to a tacit, implied authorisation. It is also important to remember that a significant aspect of the consent process is to provide *choice* for the patient, and that the outcome of that process may be either *acceptance* or *refusal* of an intervention. It is certainly not the purpose of the consent process to secure acceptance at all costs.

A further point to be noted is that the consent is an authorisation or refusal of an intervention offered to a *particular individual*, and attempts to exclude that individual from the process are likely to conflict with the principles of non-maleficence, beneficence and respect for autonomy. In other words, it is difficult to find a moral justification for obtaining consent (or refusal) from any individual other than the one to whom the intervention directly relates.

To ensure the validity of the consent process, both morally and legally, it is widely agreed that a number of elements are essential:

- competence
- information
- voluntariness.

# Competence

The notions of competence and autonomy are closely related, and it has been demonstrated that decisions about whether an individual is autonomous can be troublesome, particularly where evidence in favour of autonomy is lacking. Traditionally, standards of competence assess the ability of an individual to:

- comprehend information
- process information
- reason about the consequences of their decision.

For legal purposes, competence is either present or absent, but a decision about the competence of an individual will depend at least in part on the specific circumstances of the consent situation. For example, where an intervention carries little risk and great benefit to the individual, there may be little information for the individual to comprehend and process, and the decision may not be difficult to make. In this situation, a patient with significant impairment may nevertheless be judged to be sufficiently competent to make the decision. Where the risks and benefits of a procedure are more finely balanced, the complexity of information necessary to arrive at a decision may increase, so that even unimpaired patients may not reach the standard of competence required to make the decision. Notice, too, that a patient's competence *could* be decided by the complexity of information *made available* to them. According to this view, competence is a characteristic granted by the health worker that is beyond the control of and not intrinsic to the patient.

It is tempting to vary the threshold of competence according to the consequences of the planned intervention – for example, to demand a high level of cognitive function from patients who are making decisions with life-threatening consequences. It is easy to see how this can lead to paternalism – a health worker may decide that a particular decision carries such serious consequences that the patient cannot possibly have the ability to take that decision. In practice it is often more helpful to work from the assumption that an individual is competent until proven otherwise, and to enquire more deeply into an individual's competence to make decisions that have more serious consequences.

# Information

The information provided can determine decisions about competence, but it can also influence the consent process in other ways. The notion of fully informed consent is particularly problematic. How much information does a patient actually require to make the decision? The patient may be at a distinct disadvantage if the professional decides to withhold certain facts. The reasons for doing so may be perfectly valid – for instance, if the information is considered harmful to the patient (so-called therapeutic privilege), or the professional simply does not know the facts.

In addition to problems of disclosure, consent may be obstructed by problems of *understanding*. The distinction between understanding and competence is subtle, but Dr Smith's discussion with Freda illustrates the point well. Freda expresses the view that at her age she does not want to be treated, but this may be based on the mistaken belief that nothing can be done for older people with fractured hips. Although competent, she has misunderstood the purpose of the intervention because of a defect in the information she has been given.

A useful approach to problems of information is to address the needs of the individual, and it is important to check with the patient that they have enough information to make a decision. Where understanding is in question, it may be prudent to wait (if the urgency for the intervention is not great) until understanding is sufficient. This may mean spending considerably more time than is usual ensuring that information has been properly communicated and understood.

## Voluntariness

Healthcare decisions should be free from undue influence, and here it is helpful to refer again to the principle of respect for autonomy. The patient may be influenced by the views of the health worker, while physical or mental impairments may also restrict freedom in decision making. It should also be remembered that patient freedom may be viewed in a positive sense of *providing* all available opportunities, or in a negative sense of *not restricting* opportunity.

Let us return to the case of Jack. His expressive dysphasia considerably limited his powers of expression, and in such situations it may be easier for the patient to nod an agreement than to try to explain their reasons for refusal of a procedure. Similar arguments could be mounted for Hilda, whose profound sensory impairments limit her freedom of expression. In this sense neither patient could be said to be truly free to make decisions.

Where a patient is either unwilling or unable to provide consent, it is helpful to consider whether the individual is free from adverse influence. Such influence may be either intrinsic as a consequence of their impairments, or extrinsic as a result of coercion by others. An effort should be made to address these issues and to reduce their impact on decision making, thereby improving the validity of the consent process.

# The form of consent

When an intervention such as a surgical procedure is perceived to be of sufficient importance, the ritual of making the consent explicit may involve written documentation or a structured conversation with the patient. Where the intervention is more 'trivial', the patient's agreement may be assumed and the issue of consent then becomes tacit or implied. In the latter situation it is easy to forget about the need for consent altogether.

Making the consent process explicit in all clinical encounters could rapidly undermine the smooth and efficient administration of healthcare, to the ultimate detriment of the patient. For example, it would be ludicrous to expect written documentation of agreement for each of the tasks entailed in day-to-day care. Nevertheless, the absence of *explicit* consent does not equate to the absence of *need* for consent, and it must be remembered that consent is an issue *whenever* a medical intervention is contemplated.

# When there is no valid consent

Despite the ubiquitous nature of consent, there will be many situations in the practice of elderly care where there is simply no valid consent or refusal to be obtained. It will be clear that acceptance of this state of affairs should not be taken lightly, since due consideration must be given to factors which may be blighting the consent process. In addition, the moral validity of a consent process may be influenced by the values of health workers themselves – depending, for example, upon their particular conception of respect for autonomy or non-maleficence.

It has already been argued that there is no moral justification for obtaining consent (or refusal) from any individual other than the one to whom the intervention relates (a principle which is enshrined in English law). Nevertheless, what can be done when a patient is so impaired that it is not possible to ensure a morally (or, for that matter, legally) valid consent process? If any decision regarding health interventions is to be reached in this situation, it will have to be taken by other individuals – that is, by *surrogate* decision makers.

There are three helpful approaches to surrogate decision making:[5]

- substituted judgement
- best interests
- pure autonomy.

# Substituted judgement

The decision maker must try to decide how the patient would have decided had they been fit and able. This must entail having a knowledge of the prior beliefs and values of the patient and applying them to the present situation. Difficulty arises because it is often not possible to infer what the patient would have wanted without colouring the decision with one's own beliefs and values. Think again about Dr Smith and her patient, Harry, with dementia. She might take the view that Harry would not have wanted to be treated when he became severely demented, but this may be simply a projection of her own beliefs. For example, Harry may have believed prior to his illness that life is sacred and should be salvaged at all costs. It is thus vital when taking this approach to research thoroughly the patient's prior beliefs and values before making a decision.

# Best interests

Here the surrogate must weigh the interests that an individual might have in receiving an intervention compared with those they might have in not receiving it. Such a calculation might involve weighing the pain and suffering likely to be caused against the possible benefits of having the procedure. This will in turn depend on the nature of the procedure. For example, Dr Smith is likely to cause Harry great distress by persisting in taking blood, but the balance of interests in having the test will shift according to the reason for taking the blood. If the test is for a research project, the outcome of which is unlikely to benefit Harry, then it is unlikely to be in his best interests. However, if it is to cross-match blood for a much needed transfusion, the balance of interests shifts the other way.

# Pure autonomy

A clear and unequivocal statement by the patient about their wishes in a given situation, made while competent, is perhaps the most effective way of respecting the *prior* autonomy of an individual who has now lost their autonomy. Such an *advance directive* for healthcare decisions might be formulated in a written document such as a living will. Obvious problems with this approach ensue when the advance statement does not deal specifically with the circumstances of the present healthcare decision, or if the directive makes demands which could never be met. A directive which appoints a proxy to make certain decisions on behalf of the patient is a more practical solution. This approach both permits respect of prior autonomy and keeps the decision-making process contemporaneous.

## Consent to research

The morality of the consent process with regard to research involving older people is essentially no different from that of other healthcare interventions. Nevertheless, the emergence of research ethics committees as 'gatekeepers' in the conduct of research involving vulnerable people has ensured that the consent process for research is generally more explicit and complete than in other aspects of clinical practice.

An area of particular difficulty relates to research involving patients for whom there is no valid consent (or refusal) – for example, those with severe dementia. Surrogate decision making in this context is more problematic, since the benefits to the patient may be less obvious, unknown or even non-existent. It is unlikely that interests will weigh strongly in favour of conducting the research. It is equally unlikely that an advance directive will have anticipated the nature of future research in sufficiently specific detail to permit authorisation.

Once again, strict adherence to the principle of respect for autonomy is problematic. As a result of excluding patients who are unable to consent from research, both their condition and its treatment remain less well understood. Arguably this is just as morally unacceptable as engaging in experimentation on vulnerable adults without seeking their agreement. A way forward is to permit decisions by adults who have partial autonomy or who retain the characteristics of a person. In practice this might involve respecting the patient's *assent* to participate in research in the absence of obvious refusal. However, it is likely that research ethics committees will remain reluctant to authorise such an approach because of the potential for abuse.

## The law

A full exposition of the law of consent is beyond the scope of this chapter. The following outline is intended only to summarise the principal elements of English consent law.[6]

- Adults have a legal right to choose whether to consent to medical treatment, to refuse it, or to choose one rather than another of the treatments on offer.
- Valid consent to medical intervention provides legal defence to the health worker from civil actions in battery (unconsented touching) or negligence, and from prosecution for the crime of battery.

- For actions in battery to succeed, the plaintiff must only prove that intentional touching occurred without consent. Harm need not have occurred.
- The components of a legally valid consent are broadly that the person has capacity, has been informed about the intervention and provides the consent voluntarily.
- Adults are presumed legally competent until proven otherwise.
- The legal test of competence to consent is that the individual can comprehend and retain the relevant information, believe it, weigh the information by balancing risks and benefits, and finally arrive at a choice (which need not be a rational one).
- To avoid action in battery, a health worker need only provide information relating to the nature and purpose of the health intervention.
- To avoid action in negligence, a health worker must disclose that level of information considered to be proper by a responsible body of medical opinion.
- No adult can provide a legally effective consent (or refusal) to healthcare interventions being carried out on another adult.
- Where no consent is available because the patient lacks capacity, a health worker may legally treat the patient, so long as they act in the best interests of the patient or on the basis that the treatment is immediately necessary.

---

**Key points**

- Freely given consent to healthcare is a moral and legal imperative.
- For older people, problems may arise because a patient is unwilling or unable to provide consent, or because the carer is unwilling or unable to seek consent.
- An understanding of the moral basis of consent will help to provide solutions to consent problems which are consistent with the law.
- The moral basis of consent is derived from the principles of non-maleficence, beneficence and respect for autonomy.
- Reliance on respect for autonomy may lead to paternalism by excluding individuals who can still choose despite cognitive impairment.
- A morally and legally valid consent requires the patient to be competent, informed and voluntary.
- Consent may be explicit or tacit, but is relevant to all healthcare interventions.
- When an adult cannot provide valid consent, healthcare decisions may be justified on the basis of substituted judgement, best interests or in line with advance directives for healthcare.

# References

1   Department of Health www.doh.gov.uk/nsf/olderpeople

2   British Geriatrics Society www.bgs.org.uk

3   General Medical Council www.gmc-uk.org/standards

4   Mason JK and McCall Smith RA (2002) *Law and Medical Ethics* (6e). Butterworths, London.

5   Beauchamp TL and Childress JF (2001) *Principles of Biomedical Ethics* (5e). Oxford University Press, New York.

6   For a full account of English consent law, see Kennedy I and Grubb A (2000) *Medical Law: text with materials* (3e). Butterworths, London.

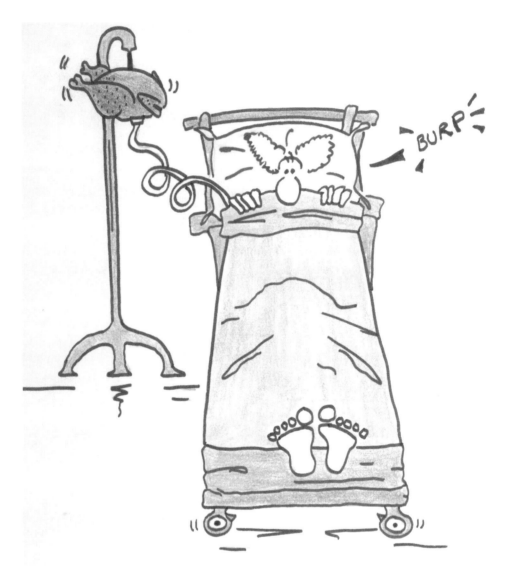

# CHAPTER 4

# Decisions on life-sustaining therapy: nutrition and fluid

## *Martin J Vernon and Olivier Gaillemin*

## Introduction

The continued receipt of food and water is fundamental to life, and to deny an individual these essential substrates seems morally indefensible. One only need conjure up media images of people starving as a result of environmental or man-made catastrophe to be reminded of the appalling consequences of malnutrition. Such images have stimulated moral debate and positive action, perhaps motivating guilt, pity or even anger that others are enduring such privation. While these examples present tangible moral dilemmas, the issues surrounding nutrition and hydration in the care of older people are perhaps less obvious, although no less important.

Older people are at risk of malnutrition for a variety of reasons, but particularly socio-economic deprivation and a higher prevalence of physical and cognitive impairments than younger adults. In one UK hospital study, nearly half of acute admissions to elderly care wards were judged to be undernourished, with one in five *severely* so. In comparison, only one in 12 general medical and one in a 100 general surgical admissions were judged to be severely undernourished.[1] Interestingly, the same study revealed that the majority of those who were undernourished on admission became more so during their hospital stay, indicating that nutrition should be high on the management agenda for ill older people.

When deciding whether or not to feed an older patient, three main strands of argument commonly emerge:

1   the scientific principles underlying the decision
2   the technical feasibility of pursuing that course of action
3   the moral principles underlying the decision.

# Scientific principles

Is there any evidence that feeding the patient will do some good? Malnutrition affects many organ systems, leading to (among other things) impairments of central nervous, cardiorespiratory and immune function, cognition and tissue repair.[2] Patients who are already challenged by pathological changes in one or more of these systems are more likely to suffer the consequences of malnutrition, leading to increased healthcare costs, morbidity and mortality. The inference of this is that supplemental nutrition may reduce the impact of some or all of these effects, speeding recovery and reducing the length of hospital stay for patients following an acute illness. This notion has been confirmed in some studies of older patients undergoing rehabilitation.[2]

Consider malnutrition resulting from dementia or a progressive neurological deficit, perhaps following loss of the desire or ability to eat. Ought we to consider artificial nutrition and hydration (ANH) to maximise the chances of recovery and reduce discomfort? Should we offer this on the grounds of palliation to all patients regardless of diagnosis or prognosis? Or are there situations where there is no benefit and only harm as a consequence of ANH?

Reasons for considering ANH in older patients range from attempts to avoid aspiration pneumonia, pressure ulcers or disability to the prevention or delay of death. However, there is mounting evidence that in some circumstances ANH may not offer the benefits intended.[3] Studies suggest that ANH is often ineffective in achieving these objectives while continuing to expose patients to potential harm.[4]

On the other hand, is there any evidence that *not* feeding a given patient is necessarily harmful? Can the absence of nutrition be beneficial in certain circumstances? For example, the feeding of dying patients can lead to unwanted or potentially harmful effects, such as increased hunger, thirst, nausea and agitation, while in some circumstances removal of hydration may *increase* patient comfort. Contrast this with a mortality rate in excess of 20% following percutaneous feeding gastrostomy placement.

When contemplating ANH it is therefore important first to consider the alternative options. For patients with advanced dementia who are experiencing swallowing difficulties, stopping anticholinergic medication, sedatives, neuroleptics or non-steroidal anti-inflammatory drugs may be sufficient to improve their nutritional intake. Other strategies include care staff education in feeding patients at risk, the use of strong flavours and finger foods, or a change in the frequency and size of meals. With such measures, survival rates with or without ANH may be no different.[5]

# Technical feasibility

Where nutritional support may be beneficial but oral feeding is impossible, what are the alternative means of accomplishing feeding? There is now a range of options at our disposal, including intravenous, nasogastric (NG), percutaneous endoscopic gastrostomy (PEG), radiographically inserted gastrostomy (RIG) or peri-oral image-guided gastrostomy (PIG). Some enteral feeding routes coupled with antibiotic protocols have made the procedure itself relatively safe, refined and effective in providing a mechanical route for feeding. However, in common with many other healthcare decisions, the availability of these techniques does not resolve the problem of whether it is *right* to employ this expertise for a particular patient.

# Moral principles

Clarifying the scientific evidence, together with an understanding of what is possible, will focus the decision-making process. Although helpful, this approach alone may not yield a morally robust solution to a clinical dilemma. Where there is no evidence of benefit from an intervention, or evidence that it might do great harm, there may be little debate. Often, however, the evidence supports several courses of action to which there are no particular technical barriers. A decision must then be made as to the right course of action.

With regard to decisions about nutrition for older patients, two morally important questions commonly arise.

1 *Should* we feed this person?
2 *Should* we *stop* feeding this person?

This chapter seeks to develop a framework for addressing these questions, and assumes that there is at least some scientific evidence in favour of the courses of action available, and that such actions are at least technically possible.

In practice, nutrition and hydration are usually provided simultaneously, and the discussion will assume this to be the case. Although some clinical situations require decisions solely about hydration, it is recommended that dilemmas relating to hydration are approached in the same way as those concerning nutrition.

# Medical treatment or basic care?

In developing a morally robust solution to the dilemma of whether or not to feed an older patient, it is necessary to consider first whether nutritional support constitutes medical therapy or basic humane care. Those who support the view that it is medical therapy have invoked the moral imperatives driving good professional practice to decide on the appropriateness of proposed treatment.[6,7] Those who adhere to the view that food is a basic necessity of life, irrespective of how it is given, have developed arguments along more humanitarian lines, free from the encumbrances of professional codes of practice.

It is interesting to note that the *procedural* nature of supplemental nutrition has a significant impact on its categorisation, and therefore on the moral arguments which surround its application. Consider the following clinical scenario.

---

**Case 1**

Gladys has been admitted to hospital with pneumonia. At the time of admission she is judged to be malnourished. She is given 'three square meals' of hospital food per day, but continues to lose weight. She is reviewed by a dietitian, who recommends supplementation and gives her cartons of liquid nutrients which she enjoys drinking. One week after admission she suffers a stroke and is unable to swallow. Nasogastric feeding is commenced and she makes good progress with rehabilitation. Unfortunately, one month later she is diagnosed with a carcinoma of the large bowel which is threatening to obstruct. The surgical team is prepared to operate, but first requests intravenous feeding to optimise her chances of recovery from the surgery.

---

At what point does the nutritional support which Gladys requires constitute medical therapy? 'Three square meals' does not appear to constitute medical therapy, since no specific procedure is involved and Gladys is free to eat normally. At first glance it would appear that her meals assume the moral status of a basic necessity of life. Nevertheless, one could present an alternative view. She is now in a medical environment which is in itself therapeutic. It is not merely the antibiotics she receives for her pneumonia which will help to restore her health, but the attentions and care of a full multi-disciplinary team including nurses, therapists, dietitian and doctors. The food she is receiving is part of this therapeutic process, and as such is subject to the same level of supervision and monitoring as other unarguably therapeutic aspects of her care.

Further support for this view arises when it becomes necessary for a nurse or other skilled professional to supervise feeding, perhaps because the patient is at risk of aspiration. Although the patient may be consuming normal food, the process of eating can be achieved safely only with the skilled supervision which is available within a therapeutic environment.

Similar arguments could be presented for the liquid nutrients Gladys is given. Such drinks are readily available outside the medical environment and could simply be viewed as a 'health food'. Alternatively, they could assume the status of treatment by contributing to the management of this patient's medical conditions which have been worsened as a result of malnutrition. This view is reinforced by the practice of prescribing these drinks, often on the advice of a dietitian.

Nasogastric and intravenous feeding appear at first glance to be more in the realm of medical therapy. They are invasive and require expertise to accomplish safely and effectively. Alternatively, one could take the view that the outcome of the process is simply to provide the patient with the food they require in order to continue living – the paraphernalia associated with feeding by these routes is a necessary but morally irrelevant encumbrance. In the legal case of Anthony Bland, a man in persistent vegetative state (PVS) who was kept alive by naso-gastric feeding, the Official Solicitor argued that ANH was distinct from medical treatment, since it was a basic necessity of life, without which he would die.[8] It was contended that doctors had a continuing duty to provide food and hydra-tion to the patient, and that to discontinue them constituted manslaughter or even murder. In response, the House of Lords took a view similar to that given with regard to the 'three square meals' given to Gladys – that the continuance of life for Anthony Bland was dependent on a comprehensive medical regime, of which nutritional support was an inseparable part. The appropriateness of continued feeding was judged on the basis that it is medical therapy, not basic care. As such it might be withdrawn or withheld like any life-prolonging treat-ment, where commencing or continuing it was not in the patient's best inter-ests. In the case of a person in PVS, doctors should make an application to Court for a declaration.

# Nutrition as medical treatment

If nutrition is assumed to be medical treatment, the process of decision making surrounding its use becomes a therapeutic decision, similar to that invoked when deciding the appropriateness of antibiotic therapy or surgery, for exam-ple. In this situation it becomes necessary to consider the objectives of therapy and the wishes of the patient concerned.

# Objectives of therapy

Before commencing a therapeutic regime, it is usual to consider the end-points one is trying to achieve, and nutritional support has an impact on at least four outcomes:

1   prolonging life
2   creating health
3   preventing disease
4   palliating terminal illness.

Before considering the moral significance of these objectives, it is important to decide whether they can be achieved. This requires consideration of two further factors.

1   Could nutrition achieve the objective for any patient?
2   Could nutrition achieve the objective for *this* patient?

It may be difficult to provide answers to these questions. Evidence in support of nutrition achieving an objective in particular circumstances may be lacking or of poor quality. Health workers may have to draw on their own experiences. The absence of high-quality evidence does not necessarily invalidate the subjective conclusions of a team of experienced professionals. It is more important that an effort is made to assess the *best available* evidence, and that the values of individuals do not contaminate such evidence. The latter situation may occur when an individual seeks to bias, suppress or ignore evidence in order to influence the final decision. The second question involves assessment of the prognosis, a process which is also imprecise and subjective. Consider, for example, the following case.

---

**Case 2**

Albert is an elderly man admitted with a stroke and unsafe swallowing. He is assessed by the stroke unit as having a 'reasonable' prognosis for good outcome. His doctor is aware of research evidence suggesting a benefit from the early use of PEG feeding following such a stroke. A request is made to the endoscopy service, but the endoscopist refuses on the basis that although the procedure is safe, the quoted evidence is of low quality. He also remarks that Albert's prognosis is 'appalling', and that he would not want a PEG tube for any relative of his with a stroke.

In this case the endoscopist is choosing to ignore evidence that the PEG tube *might* help Albert, in the absence of any clear evidence that it would definitely harm him. He is also introducing imprecise estimates of prognosis. Such views appear to be driven at least in part by the values of the endoscopist, who is opposed to PEG feeding for stroke patients in general. Failure to remain objective while assembling evidence of benefit or harm will confuse discussion of the values attached to various therapy goals. This is arguably a failure of professional duty to the patient.

Having taken care to assemble the best evidence, and to make the best estimate of prognosis, it should be possible to ascertain the likelihood of achieving various objectives. In practice, objectives will be met to a greater or lesser degree, and it is helpful to estimate where the therapy lies on the spectrum between success and failure.

For example:

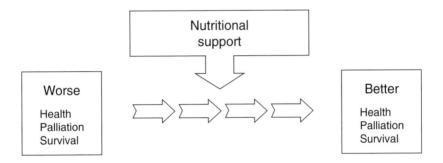

It is now necessary to decide upon the moral worth of each objective, a process which will be influenced both by the circumstances of the patient and by the professional values of those involved in the decision making. If survival is to be valued above all else, then an intervention which has any impact on improving survival will be favoured, even at the expense of poor palliation or compromised patient health. Alternatively, those who value quality of life most highly may be prepared to accept an intervention that provides palliation at the expense of reduced life expectancy.

There are several benefits of this approach. First, it makes the decision-making process explicit and provides an opportunity to separate out the practical elements of a decision (will the therapy work?) from the moral elements (which outcomes are most valued in this case?). Secondly, it may be employed by all individuals involved in the decision making, first separately and then in committee. Where moral conflict arises, it may be possible to address the problem by making explicit the values attached by individuals to the various therapeutic objectives. Thirdly, although the process requires calculations of the moral worth of various outcomes to be made, it also permits a deontological (rule-based) approach should one choose to value one particular outcome, such as the preservation of life.

# The wishes of the patient

If nutritional support has assumed the status of medical treatment, then as with any other treatment it is necessary to seek the consent of that individual before proceeding. Older patients for whom nutritional support is contemplated are often unable to participate fully in the decision making due to their illness, and difficulties arise when the wishes of the patient are not clear. One approach to this situation is outlined in Chapter 3, and the elements of the process are summarised below.

- A valid consent to treatment requires that the patient is competent, informed and voluntary.
- To be competent, a patient should be able to take in and retain information about the proposed treatment, believe it, balance the risks and benefits in their own mind and arrive at a choice.
- If the patient cannot take part in the treatment decision, by reason of incompetence, surrogates must decide in a way that is morally justifiable.

Surrogate decision making about nutritional support is not without problems. In a follow-up study of individuals who decided to accept tube feeding for their elderly incompetent relative, two-thirds were satisfied with their decision and four-fifths would do the same again.[9] Even so, almost a third of relatives in retrospect felt that the patient did not want the tube.

One way to facilitate best-interests decisions or create advance statements is to engage older people in discussions about nutritional support in advance of their requiring it. At present such discussions are not commonplace but appear acceptable to older people, can be presented in an easily comprehensible format (e.g. using vignettes) and do not provoke anxiety.[10] In one large study, only a third of competent older individuals in nursing homes would elect to have a feeding tube in the event that they suffered brain damage and were unable to eat.[11] Nevertheless, decisions by frail older people may not be durable, and discussions may have to occur repeatedly to establish a clear pattern of decision making.

# Nutrition as basic care

Where nutritional support assumes the status of basic care, decision making about its use is often driven by beliefs which surpass those employed in making a therapeutic decision. In particular, it is the values which are attached to continued comfort, well-being and ultimately life which enable the correct course of action to be decided upon.

A framework which adheres to these values is set out in the ancient Jewish ethico-legal system known as *halacha*.[12] In this system, the preservation of life takes precedence over virtually all other considerations. This stems from the belief that God has made man in his own image and in addition has given him the gift of life to be held in trust. Honouring and preserving this life is both a duty and a means of honouring God. Quality-of-life issues are of lesser importance, and only those measures that cause severe pain and suffering are to be avoided, specifically when a patient is moribund or death is imminent. In general, however, nutritional support, by whatever means, should not be refused or withdrawn, since to do so would hasten the patient's death.

Others who take a more moderate approach might view ANH as an 'extraordinary' measure which might be refused in situations where the patient is irreversibly and terminally ill. For example, patients with advanced dementia who have impaired swallowing may be considered terminally ill, given a median survival of only six months. Other moral frameworks have also employed the distinction between 'ordinary' and 'extraordinary' care in deciding about life-sustaining treatment. Care is extraordinary and therefore not obligatory if it involves great cost, pain or burden to the patient or to others, without reasonable chances of success.[13] Here the argument hinges on what one considers to be a success. If it is purely the maintenance of life, then life-sustaining care may be classed as ordinary. If success means more than this – perhaps the restoration of full health – then painful or costly care which does not meet this objective is considered extraordinary.

Opponents of this approach take the view that what is costly, painful or otherwise burdensome today might be cheap and trouble-free in the future. Indeed, the relative ease with which ANH can now be undertaken has arguably led to it becoming 'ordinary' care, whereas a decade ago it might have been considered 'extraordinary'. Others might argue that because the objectives of care determine its moral status, it is not the *care* which requires evaluation but its *endpoints*. According to this view it is less important to distinguish medical therapy from basic care, and more important to decide upon the value of the possible end-points.

The most extreme halachic view might override the values of the patient, perhaps on the grounds that no individual has the right to refuse that which gives life. Others would consider refusal only on the basis that it would prolong suffering and that otherwise every second of life is infinitely precious. In general, however, classifying nutrition as basic care removes some of the barriers to decision making which might otherwise encumber patients and their relatives when attempting to participate in a strictly *medical* decision. The complexity of medical decision making arguably makes it a less accessible process, whereas decisions based on values may be more equitable.

# Should we feed this older patient?

The approach so far has been to consider nutrition from two perspectives, namely as medical treatment or as basic care. This creates a general framework for deciding whether to start feeding a patient, which is summarised in Figure 4.1. The framework is intended only as a guide to decision making. It does not provide a comprehensive guide to all the arguments which might be mounted in favour of or against feeding, but may be used to give structure to the complex process of evaluating a particular case.

Although the question of whether or not to feed the patient is a complex one, the practical outcome of the discussion will be comparatively simple – the

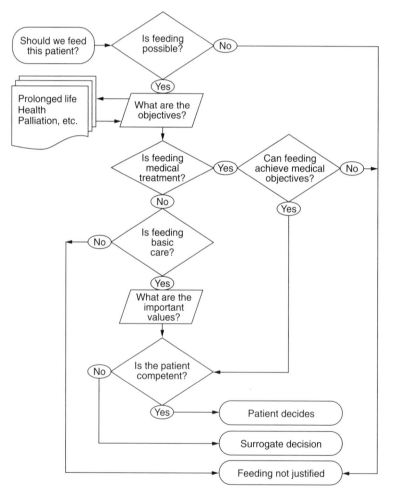

**Figure 4.1**   Decision-making scheme for initiation of feeding.

patient will or will not be fed. As with all morally important decisions, however, the outcome should be reviewed regularly to ensure that both the circumstances and the values on which the decision was based have not altered significantly over time. It has already been emphasised that a decision may be based on poor-quality evidence, and it is important to evaluate that decision in the light of new or better evidence. Where the decision was not to feed, this will involve rehearsing once more the arguments already outlined. However, once the decision has been taken to feed a patient, there are a number of additional factors to be addressed prior to discontinuing feeding.

# Should we stop feeding this older patient?

Discussions about stopping feeding will occur when it is apparent that continuing to feed is not the correct course of action. In practice, this may occur for one of three reasons:

1   patient circumstances have changed
2   the values of those involved have changed
3   issues relevant to the decision were not considered.

## Patient circumstances have changed

Where objectives of care can be met without nutritional support, perhaps because of improved patient prognosis, stopping feeding will not be problematic. Examples include recovery of swallowing following a stroke, or restoration of consciousness following overwhelming infection.

Difficulties will arise when the passage of time creates a clearer understanding of patient prognosis, leading to a change in the objectives of care. This may occur when the patient deteriorates or fails to show any signs of improvement. The following two cases illustrate these problems.

---

**Case 3**

Fred was admitted to hospital with a stroke three months ago. Because of swallowing difficulties, a PEG tube was inserted for feeding purposes. Despite comprehensive attempts at rehabilitation, he has made no progress and one week ago suffered a second stroke which has left him unconscious but otherwise clinically stable.

---

---

**Case 4**

Glenda has early dementia and was living in a residential home prior to admission. One month ago she developed septicaemia following a perforation of her colon. Following surgery to remove bowel, intravenous feeding was commenced to correct malnutrition and facilitate recovery. Despite attempts at rehabilitation, she has remained fully dependent on nursing care.

---

In the case of Fred, the objectives of feeding included maintenance of life and good functional outcome from his stroke. Recent events indicate that the latter objective is unlikely to be met, and discussion must now centre on the value attached to his continued living, together with any new objectives such as palliation of distressing symptoms. Meanwhile Glenda is unlikely to achieve functional independence, although she shows no signs of further deterioration. Here the objectives of care must alter. Rather than restoring functional independence, feeding is only likely to maintain present stability. Discussion of the appropriateness of continued feeding must therefore involve evaluation of these new or reprioritised objectives.

# The values of those involved have changed

Having gained experience of the effects of feeding over a period of time, those involved in the decision to feed may choose to alter the values they originally attached to objectives. For instance, the original decision may have been based on an overwhelming desire to maintain continued life, which has subsequently given way to the more valued objective of preventing distress. This is illustrated by the following case.

---

**Case 5**

Joyce was left with speech and swallowing difficulties following evacuation of a subdural haematoma two months ago. After discussion with her daughter and in her best interests, it was decided to insert a PEG tube to facilitate feeding. Despite attempted rehabilitation she has made no progress and remains dependent for all nursing care. She has acquired pressure sores and grimaces in pain when moved. Her daughter now feels that the need to preserve life does not justify Joyce's continued suffering.

---

When a decision has been reached by carers and relatives together, a sustained change in values of one person should prompt re-evaluation of the decision by all members of the team. This will again ensure that the basis of any new decision is explicit and based on clear objectives of care. For example, the views of Joyce's daughter may alter if she is reassured that her mother's pain can be adequately controlled and that continued feeding may help her pressure sores.

Particular difficulties may arise when the values of the *patient* become altered by the passage of time – for instance, when a patient no longer wants nutritional support. Here it is helpful to retrace the decision-making process with the patient to clarify the basis of their new decision and to evaluate their competence to do so. In certain circumstances, legal clarification may be required. This is illustrated by the following case.

---

**Case 6**

June has suffered from Parkinson's disease for five years and has become severely malnourished. Three months ago she consented to have a nasogastric tube inserted to facilitate feeding. Despite attempted rehabilitation, she has remained fully dependent and is awaiting transfer to a nursing home. She has now decided that she no longer wishes to live, and has made a refusal of further feeding via the tube.

---

Given that unconsented touching may constitute battery or assault, the implications of June's refusal for her carers are significant. Evaluating her decision making may clarify whether she is in fact competent to refuse feeding, and may elucidate the values on which she bases her refusal. This will help her carers to decide on what basis they must either respect her wishes or override her refusal.

# Issues relevant to the decision were not considered

A structured approach to decision making should ensure that all relevant issues are addressed. One safeguard to this process is to involve as many *relevant* parties as possible to permit expression of a wide range of values – for example, in the setting of a clinical ethics committee.[14] This is of particular importance when the patient cannot express their own views.

The emergence of relevant issues following a decision to feed will require the original decision to be re-evaluated and if necessary reversed, although the subsequent practical and moral difficulties may be extremely challenging.

# Killing or letting die?

No decision about nutritional support will be free from the elements of this debate, which centres on the moral equivalence of the acts which constitute killing and omissions which result in death.[15] Consider the following case.

---

**Case 7**

Jack suffered a stroke one year ago which left him unable to swallow, and a PEG tube was inserted. He now states that he wishes to die and requests that the tube be removed. This would require an endoscopic procedure, which the endoscopist refuses to undertake on the grounds that his actions would ultimately lead to Jack's death. Instead he recommends that the tube be left in place but not used. Jack's nurse argues that this has the same effect and that he does not wish to stand by and watch Jack die by his omission.

---

The endoscopist believes that an action which leads to Jack's death has more moral weight than an omission which leads to the same outcome. He could argue that removing the tube causes Jack's death, and that he is therefore killing him by agreeing to his request. He could also argue that he is assisting in Jack's suicide or even that his actions constitute active voluntary euthanasia. The nurse, on the other hand, does not draw a distinction between an act or omission, on the basis that the outcome is the same. His argument might focus on whether or not it is right for Jack to die, not on the means by which this outcome could be achieved.

One could argue that without the PEG tube, Jack's death would be inevitable, and the tube is merely a barrier to events for which Jack's carers are not responsible. Tube removal does not constitute killing him – it is simply allowing him to continue his journey towards death. Others might argue that we are obliged to remove the tube out of respect for Jack's autonomy. In this case his death may be foreseen, but it is not an *intended* effect of our actions, simply a side-effect.

Alternatively, one could argue that we have a duty to care for Jack which includes providing effective barriers to his death. If we do not prevent Jack's death then we might also decide not to prevent the deaths of others. This might place us on a 'slippery slope' towards withholding treatment for all patients who are dying. Furthermore, as carers we have a duty to care, but not to undertake activities which compromise our own moral standards. We are not obliged to do something to Jack which might lead directly to his death, even if he demands it.

There is no right or wrong solution to this dilemma, but it is important that those involved in such difficult decisions are individually comfortable with the outcome. There is no substitute to working through the arguments, guided by the frameworks outlined previously. This will not only lead to a morally robust decision, but will also facilitate discussion in those difficult cases where legal clarification is the only way forward.

# The law

In English law, the majority of cases dealing specifically with nutrition have centred on the tube feeding of individuals without their consent, or the withdrawal of tube feeding from individuals unable to express their views. Some of the key issues are summarised below.

- Food is legally identified by its chemical composition, not by its form of administration.
- Liquid food does not therefore constitute *medicine*.
- Artificial feeding does, however, form part of a *regime* which amounts to medical treatment.
- Medical treatment generally may not be administered to a competent adult without their consent.
- In the case of incompetent adults, feeding decisions should follow their best interests.
- Assessment of best interests usually includes discussion with family members.
- There is no obligation to give treatment that is futile or excessively burdensome.
- The law regards withholding or withdrawing treatment as an 'omission', not an 'act'.
- When contemplating forced feeding or withdrawal, seek legal clarification.

---

**Key points**

- A decision to artificially feed an older person requires consideration of the benefits, feasibility and morality of the proposed procedure.
- The objectives of nutritional support should be evaluated by estimating the likelihood of success.
- The wishes and values of the patient must be considered, either contemporaneously or in the form of advance statements.
- For patients who are unable to express a view, a morally robust feeding decision may emerge after wider consultation.

- Decisions to commence feeding should be reviewed in the light of changing patient circumstances or values.
- Decisions to stop or to impose feeding create complex moral problems which may require legal clarification.

# References

1   McWhirter JP and Pennington CR (1994) Incidence and recognition of malnutrition in hospital. *BMJ*. **308**: 945–8.

2   British Geriatric Society (1977, revised 2003) *Guidelines on Artificial Hydration and Nutrition in Elderly Patients*. Document G1. British Geriatric Society, London.

3   Gillick MR (2000) Rethinking the role of tube feeding in patients with advanced dementia. *NEJM*. **342**: 206–10.

4   Haddad RY and Thomas DR (2002) Enteral nutrition and enteral tube feeding. Review of the evidence. *Clin Geriatr Med*. **18**: 867–81.

5   Mitchell SL, Kiely DK and Lipsitz LA (1997) The risk factors and impact on survival of feeding tube placement in nursing home residents with severe cognitive impairment. *Arch Intern Med*. **157**: 327–32.

6   General Medical Council www.gmc-uk.org/standards

7   British Medical Association www.bma.org.uk

8   Airedale NHS Trust v Bland [1993] *1 All ER* 821.

9   McNabney MK, Beers MH and Siebens H (1994) Surrogate decision makers' satisfaction with the placement of feeding tubes in elderly patients. *J Am Geriatr Soc*. **42**: 161–8.

10  Ouslander JG, Tymchuck AJ and Krynski MD (1993) Decisions about enteral tube feeding among the elderly. *J Am Geriatr Soc*. **41**: 70–7.

11  O'Brien LA, Siegert EA, Grisso JA *et al*. (1997) Tube feeding preferences among nursing home residents. *J Gen Intern Med*. **12**: 364–71.

12  Schostack Z (1994) Jewish ethical guidelines for resuscitation and artificial nutrition and hydration of the dying elderly. *J Med Ethics*. **20**: 93–100.

13  Harris J (1985) *The Value of Life*. Routledge, London.

14  Journal of Medical Ethics http.//jme.bmjjournals.com

15  Steinbock B and Norcross A (1994) *Killing and Letting Die* (2e). Fordham, New York.

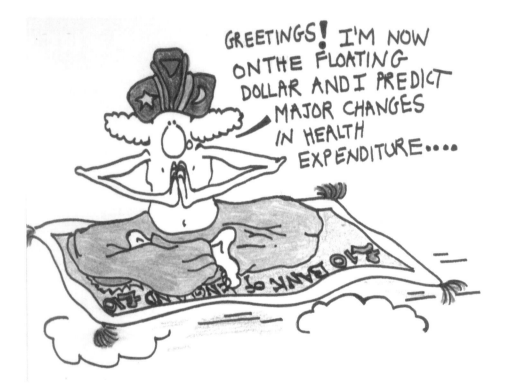

# CHAPTER 5

# Ethical issues and expenditure on health and social care

*Steven Luttrell*

## The National Health Service

In the early part of this century, medical services in the UK were spread unevenly and large numbers of poor people were not covered by the National Insurance Scheme. The National Heath Service (NHS) was established to provide equitable healthcare provision according to need, irrespective of wealth or geographical location. Over time, it became increasingly clear that comprehensive care, free at the point of delivery, was politically unsustainable. Prescription charges were introduced in 1951, and charges for ophthalmic and dental treatments were introduced thereafter. One of the most radical assaults on the provision of comprehensive care was the shedding by the NHS of substantial parts of its previously held responsibilities for continuing care. In 1982, the NHS was providing 75% of long-stay care for people aged 75 years and over. In 1996 this was reduced to just 18%. During the same time period the population of people aged 75 years and over increased by 25%.

## Health care or social care

The starting point for any discussion on the economics of healthcare must be a consideration of the meaning of the term 'healthcare'. To define certain care needs as social rather than health related transfers the funding of such services from the NHS (where, in general, costs are provided for) to social services (where, in general, costs are means tested). Although there are many areas of care which are agreed to fall clearly within the remit of the health service, there are others where this is not so obvious. For example, there has been substantial debate over which aspects of continuing care of people with disabilities should be regarded as healthcare and which should be regarded as social care. This debate was set on a legal footing in R v North and East Devon Health Authority ex part Coughlan (2000) All ER 850, which clarified the responsibilities of both health and social care services in the provision of longer-term care for people with disabilities and continuing healthcare needs.

# Principles for rationing

No matter how narrowly healthcare is defined, there remains a widespread belief that demand for services exceeds supply, and that some form of rationing or prioritisation is necessary. Rationing of healthcare is by no means a new concept. Clinicians have for many decades managed to ration their services implicitly according to unwritten rules. Broadly speaking, healthcare has in the past been rationed according to need, ability to benefit, age and desert.

## Need

The allocation of funds according to need has been a traditional function of the NHS. Initial formulas based on mortality ratios were used as proxies for need in order to redistribute funds. Empirical data have led to new formulas which are thought to be more sensitive to the influence of socio-economic factors on health, and which have been applied to the greater part of the NHS budget. However, it has been suggested that the marginal increase in equity associated with the use of the more recent formulas is probably very small, and that in future attention should be focused on the distribution of resources at local levels. Moreover, the allocation of funds according to need does not necessarily mean that such funds will confer benefit.

## Ability to benefit

Utilitarian philosophy suggests that funds should be used to provide maximum benefit. However, only a minority of interventions provided by the NHS are backed by scientific evidence that they confer benefit, and cost–benefit analysis has been applied to even fewer. Although the NHS Executive has indicated that resources should increasingly be channelled towards those interventions which are known to be effective, the paucity of data on effectiveness and cost continues to create substantial difficulties. In addition, health services have generally been slow to implement changes in practice in response to new scientific evidence of treatment benefit. With this in mind, over the past few years the NHS has established two new systems to encourage the faster implementation of clinical services and treatments where there is evidence of cost-effectiveness.

1.  The implementation of National Service Frameworks is a system aimed at ensuring that NHS services are set up in line with scientific evidence of effectiveness.
2.  Guidance from the National Institute of Clinical Excellence (NICE) is intended to steer treatment decisions in a cost-effective direction.

In practice, both of these new systems have tended to work through prioritisation (more effective practice being encouraged) rather than rationing (less effective practice being stopped). Indeed, NICE has been criticised for concentrating on new and expensive treatments, and has encountered substantial problems when it has failed to recommend the use of a new drug. For example, it faced marked hostility both from the public and from drug companies when it failed to recommend the use of beta-interferon for multiple sclerosis.

# Age

In the past, healthcare has been extensively rationed by age, and there is evidence that older people have been discriminated against with regard to renal replacement therapy, cardiological interventions and cancer treatments. A variety of reasons have been proposed to justify or explain this position.

1   It has been assumed that the needs of older people were somehow less important and that they would not, in any event, benefit from aggressive medical treatment. However, there is increasing scientific evidence that older people benefit from many medical interventions to which they would previously have been denied access (e.g. treatment of hypertension, thrombolysis for myocardial infarction, carotid artery surgery and renal replacement therapy). Increasingly it has been demonstrated that those populations at highest risk of death or complications are often the groups that benefit most from interventions. Thus in certain situations older patients, who are at a greater risk of death or morbidity than younger patients, benefit more than the latter from medical treatment.
2   It has been suggested that a strictly utilitarian method of allocating resources discriminates against older people. If it is assumed that the prime function of the NHS is to maximise health, and the 'quality-adjusted life year' (QALY) is used as a method of assessing outcome, then it becomes obvious that older people, with a shorter life expectancy, will generally rank lower on the priority list than younger people.

Harris argues against such a method of distributing resources, stating that patients want the opportunities to have the best possible combination of quantity and quality of life available to them, given their personal health status. It may be valid to use outcome measures when choosing between rival therapies, but this system should not be used for allocating resources between different groups of patients. Harris believes that it is an integral part of distributive justice that people's moral claims to resources are not diminished by who they are (how old they are, how rich or poor, powerful or weak they are) or by the quality of their lives. He argues that if the purpose of the NHS is to give people the services that they want for themselves, then they would be unlikely to choose the utilitarian approach. This argument has widespread appeal. Grimley Evans suggests that the average UK citizen sees the NHS not as a chain of grocery stores looking for the best return on its investment, but as something more akin to a motoring organisation to which a subscription is paid so that it will be there to do what the individual wants when he or she wants it.

3   It is argued by some that the older you are, the more likely you are to have had your 'fair innings', and that it would be inequitable to deny a younger person benefit in order to provide benefit for an older person.

According to one view, the fair innings argument is based on the concept of an ideal life and the notion that individuals themselves reach a point in time when they have done all that they would have wished and feel that it is appropriate that they should now die. Although this is an argument which underpins the need for a system where patient autonomy is respected, it adds little to the debate about rationing healthcare.

   According to another view, it is argued that resources should be rationed on the basis of the quality and length of life which any individual has already had. Those who have already had sufficient life of sufficient quality are of lower priority than those who have not. But how can one measure the total quality of any life and how should one decide where the cut-off point for a fair innings should be? A simpler approach has been to argue that resources should be rationed only according to the length of life which an individual has already had. This approach has popular appeal, as evidenced by the frequent media items concerning the plight of babies and children. However, it does highlight basic questions about the value that society attaches to any particular group of individuals. It might be that, despite popular appeal, to stigmatise and undervalue older people in favour of the young is detrimental to the fabric of society as a whole, especially a society that is founded on democratic principles where the value of one person is cherished as much as that of any other. The increasing political power of older people alongside the development of human rights law has done much in recent years to change society's attitude to age. Within the UK, the most explicit step to remove rationing on the basis of age was taken with the introduction of the National Service Framework for Older People, the first standard of which sets out a commitment and lists steps to remove ageism from health and social welfare decisions.

## Desert

Giving less to those who are to blame for their illness has an instant emotional appeal. However, as a method for rationing healthcare it is flawed. It is very difficult to draw up a list of those illnesses to which a voluntary choice of lifestyle has contributed. Although alcoholism and cigarette smoking cause a host of illnesses, it is arguable that neither are purely voluntary activities. If cigarette smoking is to be regarded as worthy of moral blame, then is eating an unhealthy diet to be similarly considered? Moreover, although the allocation of moral blame may fall within the responsibility of a legal system, it is questionable whether such judgements fall within the remit of a health service.

## Human Rights Act 1998

There has been only one legal case in England which has considered the implications of the Human Rights Act 1998 and patients' right to treatment. Decided in 1999 before the Act came into force in 2000, the Court of Appeal in North West Lancashire Health Authority v A, D&G concluded that a refusal to fund gender reassignment surgery did not constitute a breach of Article 3 of the Convention on Human Rights (which provides that no one should be subject to inhumane and degrading treatment), and that Article 8 (which protects respect for individuals' private lives, including their physical and psychological integrity) does not give a right to treatment. Although this case considered the convention, it is likely that a similar approach would be taken now that the Act is in force.

## International mechanisms for rationing healthcare

Some countries, such as the Netherlands, New Zealand and Sweden, have taken steps to develop explicit guidelines about allocating resources. All three countries have rejected a strictly utilitarian approach whereby services are ranked according to cost–benefit analysis.

The Swedish Commission stated that such considerations of efficiency should be limited to choices between different kinds of treatment for the same condition, and should not be invoked in the choice between claims for different services or specialities. It highlighted a number of principles which should guide all choices:

> All people have the same rights irrespective of their personal characteristics. Resources should be devoted to those in greatest need. The most vulnerable groups should be given special consideration.

The Dunning Committee in the Netherlands recommended that all claims have to pass four tests:

> Is the intervention necessary to allow the individual to function in society? Is the treatment effective? Is the treatment efficient? Could the treatment be considered a matter of individual responsibility?

The New Zealand Committee defined its principles as follows:

> The treatment should provide benefit and value for money. It should represent a fair use of resources. It should be consistent with community values.

The most adventurous project for rationing healthcare has evolved in the state of Oregon in the USA. Like every other state in the USA, it had previously provided only the poorest citizens with Medicaid and left a large percentage of the population unable to use medical services. The Commission, which heard evidence from both lay people and professionals, drew up a list of core services with a cut-off point where services at the bottom of the list would not be available. However, it would appear that the explicit prioritisation within this setting tends to result in inflation of the basic healthcare package. It has been suggested that defining a list of services to be covered must be combined with the development of clinical guidelines in order to control this.

Rudolph Klein suggests that the international principles on which there is agreement are too general to provide any assistance to those who are trying to create a core health service, and he states that rationing by such means has a trivial effect. He believes instead that the reality of rationing is the numerous day-to-day decisions made by clinicians in the light of available resources and the circumstances of the patients before them.

The UK Government has not taken steps to define in explicit terms the principles which should be used to ration healthcare, appearing to rely instead on the development of policy from various NHS quality initiatives in combination with the accumulated decisions of healthcare trusts and individual clinicians. Much media and political attention has been paid to the fact that treatment options appear to differ from one part of the country to another. The mechanisms which have been established to counteract this include the development of national standards through a combination of National Service Frameworks and guidance set out by the National Institute for Clinical Excellence. At the same time the Government has been keen to devolve responsibility for resource allocation to a local level, and responsibility for the allocation of over 70% of the NHS budget now rests with primary care trusts. The implications of the inevitable tensions which are created by a system which sets national standards but expects local financial responsibility are not yet clear, nor is it clear whether the systems that have been established are sufficiently robust to provide a fair method of allocating resources.

---

**Key points**

- The NHS was founded on the principle that it would provide an equitable system of healthcare.
- Narrowing the remit of the NHS has been used as a political method for reducing healthcare expenditure.
- Even if healthcare is defined in narrow terms, there appears to be a substantial financial gap between supply and demand.
- Rationing has traditionally been implicit and based on a variety of factors, such as age, desert, need and ability to benefit.
- A number of countries have attempted to make explicit the principles which should be used in rationing healthcare.
- In the UK, systems have been introduced over the past few years in order to steer service delivery along lines which are backed by evidence of effectiveness.
- There is little international agreement about the most effective and fair methods of resource allocation.

---

# Further reading

- Department of Health HSC 2001/015: LAC (2001) 18 NHS continuing health care NHS and local council's responsibilities.

- Department of Health (2001) *National Service Framework for Older People*. Department of Health, London.

- Doyal L (1997) The rationing debate. Rationing within the NHS should be explicit: the case for. *BMJ.* **314**: 1114.

- Grimley Evans J (1993) Health rationing and elderly people. In: M Turnbridge (ed.) *Rationing of Health Care in Medicine*. Royal College of Physicians, London.

- Grimley Evans J (1997) Rationing healthcare by age. The case against. *BMJ*. **314**: 822–5.

- Ham C (1998) Retracing the Oregon trail: the experience of rationing and the Oregon health plan. *BMJ*. **316**: 1965–9.

- Harris J (1991) Unprincipled QALYs: a response to Cubbon. *J Med Ethics*. **17**: 185–8.

- Harris J (1997) Maximising the health of the whole community. The case against: what the principal objective of the NHS should really be. *BMJ*. **314**: 669–72.

- House of Commons Health Committee (1995) *Priority Setting in the NHS: purchasing. Volume 1*. HMSO, London.

- Klein R (1997) Defining a package of healthcare services the NHS is responsible for. The case against. *BMJ*. **314**: 506–9.

- Maynard A (1995) Distributing healthcare rationing and the role of the physician in the United Kingdom National Health Service. In: A Grubb and MJ Mehlman (eds) *Justice and Health Care: comparative perspectives*. John Wiley & Sons, Chichester.

- New B, on behalf of the Rationing Agenda Group (1996) The rationing agenda in the NHS. *BMJ*. **312**: 1593–601.

- Sheldon T (1997) Formula fever: allocating resources in the NHS. *BMJ*. **315**: 964.

- Smith R (2000) The failings of NICE. *BMJ*. **321**: 1363–4.

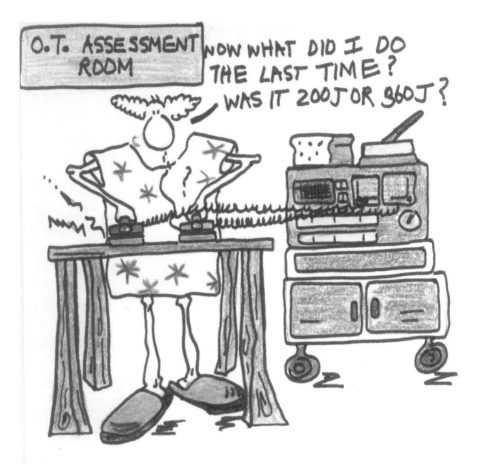

# CHAPTER 6

# Cardiopulmonary resuscitation

*Rachel Powis, Kevin Stewart and Gurcharan S Rai*

## Introduction

Cardiopulmonary resuscitation (CPR) is routinely attempted when hospital inpatients suffer cardiac arrest, unless a specific decision is made in advance to withhold it. However, such 'do not attempt resuscitation' (DNAR) decisions can be controversial. In the UK, there has been considerable press and public concern about DNAR decisions following several high-profile cases, and there have been demands for more openness and transparency in the decision-making process.

The response of professional bodies, namely the British Medical Association (BMA) and the Royal College of Nursing with the Resuscitation Council (UK), has been to update and improve the guidelines on DNAR decision making. These were published in January 2002 and have incorporated many of the provisions of the Human Rights Act which came into force in the UK in October 2000.

## The guidelines on CPR

The articles of the Human Rights Act which may pertain to decision making about resuscitation include the following:

- Article 2 – the right to life
- Article 3 – the right to freedom from inhuman or degrading treatment
- Article 8 – the right to respect for privacy and family life
- Article 10 – the right to hold opinions and receive information
- Article 14 – the right to be free from discriminatory practices (e.g. ageism).

The new guidelines incorporate several important changes, some of which have been included in recognition of the provisions of the Human Rights Act. They recognise that:

1 the goal of medicine is not to prolong life at all costs with no regard to its quality or burden of treatment on the patient
2 a competent patient has the right to accept or refuse resuscitation after he or she has been fully informed of its benefits and risks
3 the consultant or general practitioner should always be prepared to discuss DNAR decisions with competent patients
4 consultants and the general practitioner should usually consult other professionals
5 under the Human Rights Act, relatives and carers have the right to information with the consent of the competent patient. The role of relatives and carers is to help the doctor in decision making and to reflect what a competent patient would want in the circumstances. They do not have the right to demand or reject resuscitation or a DNAR order
6 the overall responsibility for decisions about CPR and DNAR rests with the consultant or general practitioner in charge of the patient's care, and this may lead to dispute with the other professionals in the multi-disciplinary team.

Some of the recommendations in the latest guidelines are likely to lead to practical difficulties. For example, it is recommended that DNAR decisions should usually be discussed with competent patients (unless there is a clear indication that the patient does not want this, or that it would be harmful), and that DNAR orders cannot be written for such patients without their agreement. This is the case even if the likelihood of CPR succeeding is thought to be so low as to be considered medically 'futile', although many doctors will traditionally have made decisions on this basis without feeling the need to obtain the patient's consent. Article 8 of the Human Rights Act recognises the place of relatives and friends, and the guidelines recommend that they should usually be involved in decisions and informed about them, bearing in mind the need to maintain proper regard for patient confidentiality. It is also suggested that 'senior experienced doctors' should make decisions, but the practicalities of this may prove difficult.

# Making a DNAR decision

## When should a DNAR decision be made and on which patients?

Only a minority of patients who are admitted acutely to hospital will undergo a CPR attempt; most are discharged alive. However, predicting which patients will potentially require CPR is difficult, and this leads to some clinicians attempting to make resuscitation decisions for all patients who are admitted to hospital acutely. Yet this may not be practicable in future, with an increasingly complex decision-making process and time pressures on staff. We know that most of those patients who survive CPR arrest within the first couple of days of hospital admission, but at this time many patients may be too ill to be involved in decision making.

It is considered appropriate to make a DNAR decision in the following five circumstances:

1   where the clinical outcome, including the likelihood of successfully starting the patient's heart and breathing, is poor
2   where CPR is not in accord with the recorded, sustained wishes of the patient who is mentally competent
3   where successful CPR is likely to be followed by a length and quality of life which would be unacceptable to the patient
4   where the patient already has a poor quality of life and does not wish to have his or her life prolonged
5   where the patient is in the terminal phase of an illness.

## Who should make the decision?

The guidelines recommend that 'senior experienced doctors' should take responsibility for decision making. In hospital practice this is likely to mean those at consultant or specialist registrar level, or those with similar experience. It seems unlikely that it would be acceptable for doctors at house-officer or senior-house-officer level to routinely make decisions on their own, especially since some of the recent adverse publicity has involved doctors at this level. However, in some circumstances it may be acceptable for such junior staff to make decisions. For example, if a terminally ill patient is admitted to hospital and family members request a DNAR decision from a junior doctor at a time when a senior colleague is not readily available, it seems reasonable to comply with this. However, if there is doubt or disagreement about decisions or if junior members of staff feel unable to make a decision in the absence of senior colleagues, full active treatment should be given until the situation is resolved.

## Discussion with the patient and his or her family

In the USA, all DNAR orders require the permission of the patient or a surrogate, whereas in the UK the decision has traditionally been left to the doctor. However, the new guidelines recommend that all DNAR orders should be discussed with competent patients, unless they indicate that they do not want to discuss them. If a doctor feels that discussion is likely to be harmful (i.e. cause anxiety and distress), this may be a justification for avoiding it in some cases, but this must be documented clearly in the medical records.

General discussion of CPR should focus on the risks and benefits of CPR for the individual, with the doctor giving a realistic estimate of the chances of survival, and should address the patient's perception of his or her quality of life and the appropriateness of any life-saving or life-sustaining treatment. The decision here will rest much more with the patient than with anyone else. If the patient is a good candidate for CPR, the doctor must also respect the patient's wishes, even if these are in opposition to his or her own.

In cases where discussion with the patient is likely to be harmful, or if the patient is too ill to express a view, the doctor may approach the family, particularly if the relatives have raised such issues. Under these circumstances the aim of discussion should be to discover the prior wishes of the patient, his or her religious beliefs, and his or her attitude to the anticipated treatment and to continued life itself. A suggested format of one of the questions is 'What do you think he/she would have liked if he/she had been able to tell us?'. Relatives and friends are being asked to reflect what the patient would have wanted in the circumstances, not what they themselves think should be done or what they would want for themselves in similar circumstances. However, the views of relatives should not be regarded as overriding, as the doctor's primary responsibility is to the patient, and circumstances are conceivable in which the patient's best interests and the relatives' views could be at variance.

When eliciting the views of the patient and their family it is important to ensure that they possess reasonable knowledge of CPR and the likely success of the procedure. If they do not possess such knowledge, it is important for the physician to provide this information in simple language so that an elderly person and their relatives are able to understand it and use it in reaching a decision about CPR.

# Discussion with incompetent patients

In order to be ethically and legally competent to consent to treatment, the patient should be able to:

1 understand a simple explanation of a proposed treatment, its outcome and complications
2 reason consistently about specific goals of treatment
3 choose to act on the basis of such reasoning and communicate his or her choice
4 understand the consequences of his or her choice.

Legally and ethically a competent person can make any and all decisions about treatment, and the doctor's primary duty is the care of the patient. The patient can refuse or accept treatment that overrides objections from the family.

If the patient is not competent to participate in discussion, and has not left clear instruction in the form of a living will or an advance directive, then the doctor should consult other professionals involved in the care of the patient and his or her relatives or carers. After discussion, the doctor has the responsibility for making a decision that is considered to be in the best interests of the patient.

# Patients who become mentally incompetent as a result of acute illness after they have made a decision

If a patient becomes incompetent after they have made a decision, then their original decision stands provided that the circumstances which have arisen are as envisaged by the patient when they made the decision.

## Role of the relatives in discussion

Relatives will often insist that they have the right not only to information about the patient's illness but also to be involved in decisions about treatment, including resuscitation. Until recently, relatives had no right to demand such action from a doctor. However, Article 8 of the Human Rights Act, which recognises the right to private and family life, gives them the right to be involved in the discussion, with the full knowledge and consent of the competent patient. Although it is not possible to nominate a proxy decision maker in England, Wales and Northern Ireland, this can be done in Scotland.

## Conflict between patients and their relatives

Conflict between patients and their relatives can arise under several circumstances:

1   if a competent patient refuses to give permission to the doctor to discuss his or her medical condition and treatment options – under these circumstances, the patient's rights override those of the relatives

2   if the decision made by the competent patient is different to that suggested by the relatives – under these circumstances, the physician should facilitate a discussion between them with the aim of reaching a decision that has been made by the patient

3   if the relatives question the patient's competency, then doctors should be able to defend their assessment of competence.

# When the success of CPR is considered to be poor

Until recently the concept of 'medical futility' has been used in DNAR decisions. Ethically and legally it was accepted that if the treatment offers little benefit it need not be offered to the patient, and under these circumstances the patient need not be involved in the discussion.

However, the new guidelines reject the concept of futility and recognise the right of the individual to be involved in decisions about CPR, even when there is a very small chance of it succeeding. This reflects the provision of the Human Rights Act which recognises patients' right to information about their care, rather than simply asking for their consent to treatment which has already been decided on.

# Legal aspects of CPR decision making

1   There is no specific law covering CPR.

2   If we include CPR as part of treatment, a competent patient has a right to consent to it or refuse consent to it.

3   In the case of an incompetent patient, the doctor should discuss the benefits and risks of CPR with close relatives/carers and other staff and reach a decision based on what would be in the best interest of the patient. If the joint discussion reaches the conclusion that CPR would be inappropriate, as it will add nothing to the patient's well-being as a person, then the doctor is not required to offer it.

4   Under the Human Rights Act 1998 a competent patient has the right to refuse a DNAR decision made by a physician and ask him or her not to document it in the medical records. Under these circumstances, the physician is obliged to follow this decision provided that there is a chance that resuscitation will lead to restoration of the patient's pulse and breathing.

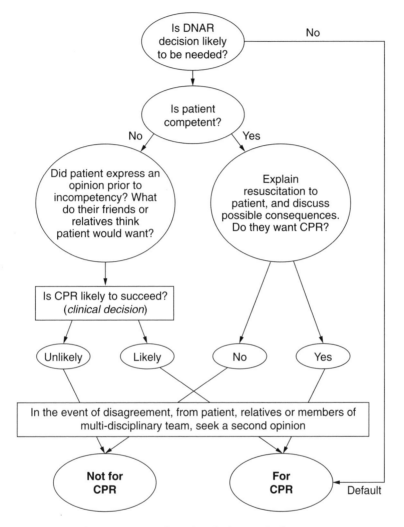

**Figure 6.1**  Suggested resuscitation algorithm for hospital admission.

---

**Case 1**

Mrs A, aged 84 years, was admitted to hospital with intracerebral bleeding following a fall. She had a past history of manic-depressive illness and required supervision from her husband for basic activities of daily living. At the time of admission she had a Glasgow Coma Score of 9/15, and had spontaneous movement in the left arm and left leg but no movements in the right leg and right arm and bilateral plantar extensor responses. The duty medical registrar who assessed Mrs A made a DNAR decision on the grounds that CPR was unlikely to be successful. However, when he discussed this with Mrs A's husband, who was very close to his wife, and her daughter, they demanded that she should be resuscitated in the event of a cardiorespiratory arrest. The doctor pointed out the fact that, in his view, Mrs A would not survive resuscitation. As a stalemate was reached, another meeting was organised for the next day and on this occasion the family were again informed that (1) resuscitation would be unsuccessful and (2) a DNAR decision would not lead to Mrs A being deprived of any other treatment. In fact, she went on to have a PEG tube inserted and received two courses of antibiotics for pneumonia.

Comments
1   It is important to point out to the patient's family or carers as well as other professionals that a DNAR decision does not mean automatic denial of other appropriate treatment.
2   Although it is important to involve the family in decision making, particularly when the patient is incapable of making a decision for him- or herself, it is equally important to note that the doctor's primary responsibility is to the patient. If the relatives' views and what would be in the patient's best interest are at variance, the doctor must make a decision that is in the best interest of the patient, after an assessment of the benefits, burdens and risks.

Case 2

An 84-year-old woman with longstanding rheumatoid arthritis, who required a considerable amount of aid and support from the community services in order to live at home, was admitted with a one-week history of nausea and vomiting. In addition to rheumatoid arthritis, she had a past history of left hip replacement, bilateral knee replacements and ischaemic heart disease. The doctors who admitted her concluded that it would be difficult to resuscitate her successfully should she have a cardiorespiratory arrest, and recorded DNAR in her notes. They did not discuss this with the patient.

Comments
Previous guidelines would suggest that although it is important to involve the patient in CPR decision making, discussion need not take place if the

CPR is likely to be futile. Futility as a rationale for CPR decision making is rejected by the new guidelines, which take into account the articles under the Human Rights Act 1998. Doctors should have a detailed discussion of the reasons for a possible DNAR order, a description of the processes and a realistic view of the possible outcomes. Although doctors cannot be required to give treatment that is contrary to their clinical judgement, they should whenever possible respect the patient's wishes to receive treatment which has only a small chance of success or benefit.

# Further reading

- British Medical Association (2000) *The Impact of the Human Rights Act 1998 on Medical Decision Making*. British Medical Association, London.

- British Medical Association (2002) *Decisions Relating to Cardiopulmonary Resuscitation. A joint statement from the British Medical Association, the Resuscitation Council (UK) and the Royal College of Nursing*. British Medical Association, London.

- General Medical Council (2002) *Withholding and Withdrawing Life-Sustaining Treatments: good practice in decision making*. General Medical Council, London.

- O'Keefe S, Redhan C, Keane P and Daly K (1991) Age and other determinants of survival after in-hospital cardiopulmonary resuscitation. *Q J Med*. **81**: 1005–10.

- Stewart K, Wagg W and Kiniorns M (1996) When can elderly patients be excluded from discussing resuscitation? *J R Coll Physicians Lond*. **30**: 133–5.

- Stewart K, Claire S and Rai GS (2003) Where now with Do Not Attempt Resuscitation decisions? *Age & Ageing*. **32**: 143–8.

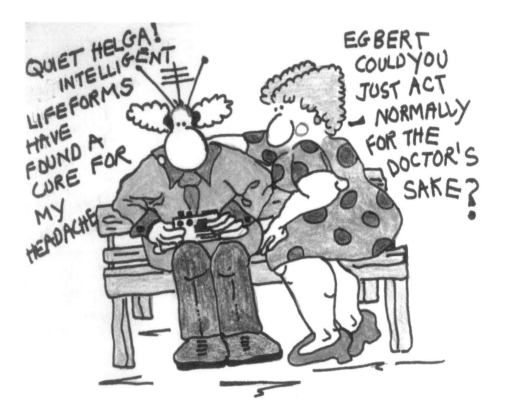

# CHAPTER 7

# Mental incapacity and best interests

## *Steven Luttrell*

The right of a mentally competent adult to refuse medical or any other intervention is enshrined in the common law in the UK and reinforced by the Human Rights Act 1998, which incorporates the European Convention on Human Rights into domestic law. A person may refuse treatment for reasons which are 'rational, irrational or for no reason', and a doctor may be liable for assault or battery or for breach of Article 8* of the Convention on Human Rights if they touch a person contrary to his or her wishes. However, if the person is mentally incapable, whether temporarily or permanently, the doctor has a duty to act in his or her best interests.

A decision on mental capacity is ultimately a question of law for a court to decide. However, most decisions about mental capacity to make decisions about medical treatment never reach the hands of lawyers, and are undertaken by the treating doctor.

Mental incapacity is a significant issue for doctors who provide healthcare for older people, due to the high prevalence of both dementia and delirium.

## Legal rules for assessing mental capacity for medical decisions

The present legal rules for the assessment of mental capacity vary according to the decision undertaken. The rules governing capacity to make decisions about medical treatments were initially set out in 'Re C' (1994), a case in which the High Court was asked to decide whether a schizophrenic patient

---

* Article 8 of the Human Rights Act is the right to private and family life, and also incorporates the right to protect the physical integrity of a person.

from Broadmoor Hospital was mentally competent to refuse amputation of a gangrenous leg. It was stated that an adult has the capacity to refuse medical treatment if he or she can:

1  understand and retain the information relevant to the decision in question
2  believe that information
3  weigh that information in the balance to arrive at a choice.

Although useful, it has been suggested that this test is not quite accurate in that a person is not necessarily mentally incapable simply because he or she does not believe his or her doctor.

The issue of how to determine mental capacity was further reviewed by both the Law Commission and the Scottish Law Commission in their reports on mental incapacity, and by the Court of Appeal in 'Re MB' (1997), a case concerning a young pregnant woman. The conclusions of the reports are broadly similar, and the capacity test in 'Re MB' is as follows.

> A person lacks capacity if some impairment or disturbance of mental function renders the person unable to make a decision whether to consent to or to refuse treatment. That inability will occur when:
>
> (a)  the person is unable to comprehend and retain the information which is material to the decision, especially as to the likely consequences of having or not having the treatment in question;
> (b)  the person is unable to use the information and weigh it in the balance as part of the process of arriving at a decision.

The decision about mental capacity will vary according to the gravity of the decision. The more serious the decision, the greater the capacity required.

## Assessing mental capacity

In cases where mental capacity is severely impaired, the assessment will often be straightforward. However, where impairment is mild or moderate, the assessment may be difficult. In such cases you should make a comprehensive examination of mental function, having regard to the fact that an abnormality in behaviour, language function, mood, thought, perception, insight, cognition, memory, intelligence or orientation may result in an inability to make decisions, thereby rendering the person mentally incapable.

Evidence from other members of the multi-disciplinary team, especially nursing and therapy colleagues, and also from the patient's relatives or friends, may be helpful in coming to a decision.

The need to seek an independent opinion in difficult cases was set out in guidance in 'St George's Healthcare NHS Trust v S' (1998), where it was stated by the Court of Appeal that:

The authority should identify as soon as possible whether there is concern about a patient's competence to consent to or refuse treatment. If the capacity of the patient is seriously in doubt it should be assessed as a matter of priority. In many such cases, the patient's general practitioner or other responsible doctor may be sufficiently qualified to make the necessary assessment, but in complex cases involving difficult issues about the future health and well-being or even the life of the patient, the issue of capacity should be examined by an independent psychiatrist, ideally one approved under Section 12(2) of the Mental Health Act. If following this assessment there remains serious doubt about the person's competence and the seriousness or complexity of the issues in the particular case may require involvement of the court, the psychiatrist should further consider whether the patient is incapable by reason of mental disorder of maintaining her property or affairs. If so, the patient may be unable to instruct a solicitor and will require a guardian *ad litem* in any court proceedings. The authority should seek legal advice as quickly as possible.

It is important to realise that the assessment of mental capacity is specific to the decision being undertaken. A person with borderline capacity may be able to make simple decisions concerning treatment of a straightforward nature, but unable to make a decision on a more complex issue. Furthermore, mental capacity may vary from time to time.

The assessing doctor should take the following steps to minimise those reversible factors which reduce capacity.

1   Treatable medical conditions which affect mental capacity (e.g. acute confusion and depression) should be addressed, and if possible the assessment should be delayed until capacity is maximal.
2   Sensory impairments should be corrected if possible.
3   Care should be taken to choose the best location and time for the assessment.
4   A decision should be reached as to whether the presence of a friend, relative or interpreter would be helpful.

The question 'Is the person mentally incapable?' should be answered on the balance of probabilities (i.e. 'Is it more probable than not that the patient lacks the required mental capacity?'). This is a less stringent test than the 'beyond reasonable doubt' test that is used in criminal law. Everyone is presumed to be mentally capable until proved otherwise. However, once it is proved that a person is mentally incapable there is a presumption that this continues until the contrary is established.

The patient should be informed about the nature of the assessment, its implications and the process by which decisions are made. During the assessment the
doctor should avoid asking leading questions.

# Making decisions for a mentally incapable adult

Patients who are mentally incapable should be treated in their best interests.
Under English law no other person can give or withhold consent for a mentally
incapable adult. The legal issues relating to best-interests decisions are most
clearly set out in Re S (sterilisation: patient's best interests) (2000) 2 FLR 389,[1]
where it was proposed that a two-stage test should be applied. The first stage is
the application of the 'Bolam test'. This is a legal test applied to negligence law
which states that the treatment will be lawful if it accords with practice
accepted as proper by a responsible body of medical opinion. It was recognised
that this approach may provide the patient with a number of different treatment
options. For mentally capable patients, the doctor would proceed to explain the
range of alternatives, concentrating on those features of advantage and disadvantage most relevant to the patient's needs and circumstances. This step is
not possible for a mentally incapable patient, and in these circumstances the
second step is to make a choice on behalf of the person. LJ Thorpe explained
this second step by stating:

> In deciding what is best for the disabled patient the judge must have regard
> to the patient's welfare as the paramount consideration. That embraces
> issues far wider than the medical. Indeed, it would be undesirable and prob-
> ably impossible to set bounds on what is relevant to a welfare determina-
> tion. In my opinion, Bolam has no contribution to make to this second and
> determinative stage of the judicial decision.

Although LJ Thorpe stated that it would be undesirable to set bounds on those
factors which are relevant to a welfare decision, previous judicial decisions on
best interests have indicated that factors such as steps to improve or prevent
deterioration in health, the invasiveness of the treatment, the indignity to
which a person has to be subjected, and the person's quality of life following
treatment might all be relevant to best-interests decisions.

# Law reform

In its 1995 report on mental incapacity, the Law Commission made a number
of recommendations to clarify and add to the law with respect to mentally

incapable adults. Following a period of consultation, many of these recommendations are now reflected in the recently published (June 2003) draft Mental Incapacity Bill for England and Wales, issued by the Secretary of State for Constitutional Affairs.

1   The draft bill sets out a test for mental incapacity which broadly follows that set out in 'Re MB'.
2   Although the present common law enables another person to make a decision on behalf of a mentally incapable adult, this aspect of the law is not well understood, and the bill clarifies this, stating that it will be lawful for a person to do an act when providing any form of care for another person (P) if either P is mentally incapable or the person reasonably believes P to be mentally incapable and in all the circumstances it is reasonable for the person to do the act.
3   The bill also sets out a number of factors to which a person must have regard when making decisions for a mentally incapable adult. These factors include the following:
    ● whether the person is likely to have capacity in relation to the matter in question in the future
    ● the need to permit and encourage the person to participate, or to improve his ability to participate, as fully as possible in any act done for and any decision affecting him
    ● so far as is ascertainable, (i) the person's past and present wishes and feelings and (ii) the factors which he would consider if he were able to do so
    ● if it is practicable and appropriate to consult them, the views of (i) any person named by the person as someone to be consulted on the matter in question or on matters of that kind, (ii) any person engaged in caring for him or interested in his welfare, (iii) any donee of a lasting power of attorney granted by him, (iv) any deputy appointed for him by the court, as to his past and present wishes and feeling and the factors he would consider if he were able to do so
    ● whether the purpose for which any act or decision is needed can be as effectively achieved in a way less restrictive of his freedom of action.
4   The bill makes provision for the creation of a new form of power of attorney that will allow a person to appoint an attorney on his or her behalf if he or she should lose capacity in the future. This 'lasting power of attorney' will apply to welfare (including healthcare) and financial decisions, a remit which is much wider than the current enduring power-of-attorney system.

The Hague Convention on the International Protection of Adults 2000 provides international protection for adults who are unable to protect their own interests. The convention highlights international co-operation in these cases, and aims to avoid conflict between the legal systems of different member states.

Scotland has incorporated the code into its Adults with Incapacity Act, and it is intended that the code will be similarly incorporated into the Mental Incapacity Bill for England and Wales.

# The Mental Health Acts

Mental capacity is not relevant to the working of the Mental Health Act 1983 in England and Wales and the Mental Health (Scotland) Act 1984. The various sections of these acts are not framed in terms of mental incapacity, but in terms of mental illness and the interests of the patient's health and safety and the protection of others. If applicable, the acts allow the treatment of mental illness without the consent of the person. Although it is not possible to treat coexisting physical illness, it is possible to treat physical illness which is a cause or a consequence of the mental illness. Thus it is possible to force-feed a patient with anorexia under the act, whereas it is not possible to amputate a gangrenous leg simply because the patient has schizophrenia.

# Medical research

The assessment of mental capacity to participate in research is identical to that for medical treatment. However, as a matter of good practice, all research – whether it involves mentally capable or incapable adults – should be approved by a research ethics committee.

The enrolment of mentally incapable patients into research studies is a controversial area, and the law is unclear. Research can be broadly categorised as therapeutic or non-therapeutic. In the case of therapeutic research there is an intention to benefit the patient (e.g. most randomised controlled trials). However, non-therapeutic research offers no direct benefit to the individual patient, but may provide valuable information that is helpful to the treatment of others (e.g. studies investigating the aetiology or pathological aspects of disease).

The Law Commission suggested that, in the case of therapeutic research, the best-interests test governs decisions as to whether the patient should participate. However, in the case of non-therapeutic research it is argued that participation cannot be justified under this test, as the individual will not incur any direct benefit. If this is the case, such participation is unlawful and may constitute a battery. The Law Commission acknowledged the usefulness of non-therapeutic research and recommended a change to the law to make such research lawful if certain criteria were fulfilled, namely:

1 the research relates to the condition from which the patient suffers
2 the same knowledge cannot be gained from research limited to those capable of consenting
3 the procedures involve minimal risk and invasiveness.

However, these proposals have not been incorporated into the proposed Mental Incapacity Bill.

# Mental capacity for non-medical decisions

The law relating to non-medical decisions and mental incapacity is generally similar to that for medical decisions. At present in England and Wales there is a variety of slightly different common law tests for determining mental capacity relating to different decisions (i.e. there is a specific test for mental capacity to make a will, to enter into a contract, to marry, etc.). The draft Mental Incapacity Bill provides one uniform test for mental capacity and a single system of law governing the way in which decisions should be made for a mentally incapable adult, whether they be related to health, social welfare or finance. It is a welcome replacement for the current confusing array of common law options.

---

**Key points**

- The right of a mentally capable adult to refuse medical or any other intervention is enshrined in UK law.
- A person is mentally incapable if he is unable by reason of a mental disability to make a decision for himself on the matter in question, or is unable to communicate his decision.
- A person is unable to make a decision if he is unable to understand or retain the information (in broad terms and simple language) relevant to the decision, or is unable to make a decision based on that information.
- If a person is mentally incapable, the decision must be made in that person's best interests.
- In reaching a best-interests decision you should have regard to the previous wishes and feelings of the person and those factors that the person would consider if able to do so. You should also consider the views of others whom it is appropriate and practical to consult.
- The assessment of mental capacity to participate in research is identical to that for medical treatment.

# Reference

1   Re S (sterilisation: patient's best interests) (2000) 2 FLR 389.

# Further reading

- An overview of the draft Mental Incapacity Bill; www.lcd.gov.uk/menincap/overview. htm

- St George's Healthcare NHS Trust v S (1998) 3 All ER 673.

- Re MB (1997) 2 FLR 426.

- Re C (adult: refusal of treatment) (1994) 1 WLR 290.

- British Medical Association (1995) *Assessment of Mental Capacity: guidelines for doctors and lawyers. A report of the British Medical Association and the Law Society.* British Medical Association, London.

- The Law Commission (1995) *Mental Incapacity.* HMSO, London.

- Hoggett B (1996) *Mental Health Law* (4e). Sweet & Maxwell, London.

- Scottish Law Commission (1995) *Report on Incapable Adults.* HMSO, Edinburgh.

---

**Case 1**

Mrs Smith is an older woman with dementia. She was admitted to hospital following a period of increased confusion associated with a chest infection. At the time of admission she was disorientated, and she was assessed by the admitting doctor as incapable of making a decision about admission to hospital or treatment. Her close friend, Mrs Singh, indicated that she enjoyed her life and had given no indication that she did not wish to receive treatment in these circumstances. To the best of her knowledge Mrs Smith had not completed a living will. Mrs Smith's sister was on holiday and was not contactable. Mrs Smith was admitted to hospital and her chest infection was treated in her best interests.

**Comment**
Although she underwent a period of rehabilitation, Mrs Smith never regained her previous level of independence, and many members of the multi-disciplinary team had concerns about her safety should she return home. She was further assessed and found to be unable to appreciate the risks associated with living in her own home and incapable of making a decision about returning to live there. However, her close friend, Mrs Singh, stated that she had previously indicated to her on many occasions

---

both prior to and after her diagnosis of dementia that if at all possible she wanted to remain in her own home and did not want to live in a nursing home. Once this view was confirmed by Mrs Smith's sister, it was agreed that Mrs Smith would have accepted some risks in order to remain in her own home, and that in the present circumstances it would be in her best interests to return home. All reasonable steps were taken to reduce these risks by means of home adaptations and home care.

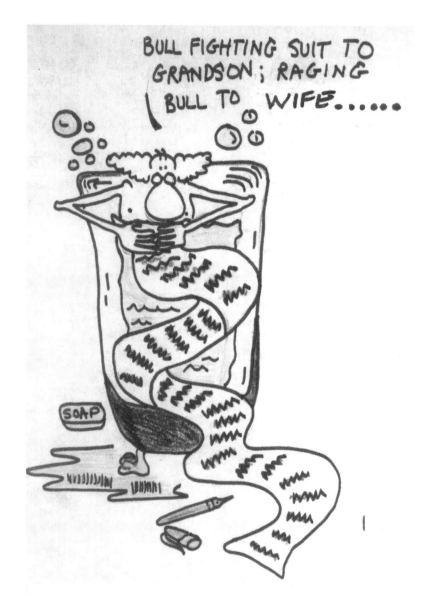

# CHAPTER 8

# Advance directives

## *Donald Portsmouth*

An advance directive, otherwise known as a living will,[1] is a statement of treatment preferences that indicates a person's wishes should the capacity for decision making be lost in the future. Based on the principle of autonomy, it aims to project this forward into possible future mental incapacity.

In UK law, no one has the right to give consent for the treatment of another adult (the situation in Scotland is somewhat different[2]). Faced with a patient who is unable to participate in decision making and thus unable to give consent, a doctor acts under his or her 'duty of care' in what is considered the patient's 'best interests'. In practice, this can leave the medical team in doubt as to the best course of action to take in the circumstances of a gravely ill elderly patient. Discussion with close relatives is of course part of good practice, but their views may conflict with each other and also with the medical view of what is a reasonable and acceptable course of action.

There is a popular notion that medicine may sometimes go too far and preserve life at all costs by applying aggressive treatment. In common with society's desire to control events in our own lives, it seems only reasonable that we should have the right to control what may be the most important decisions of all, namely the treatment that we wish to receive when seriously ill.

The principle of 'informed consent' to treatment is firmly established in medical ethics and clinical practice, although the law in the UK does not recognise the concept as in the USA. It is better to use the term 'valid consent' as authorising treatment. To treat a competent patient without their consent can be held to be an assault on them.[3] In practice, however, such consent can be assumed by a patient's compliance. This depends on providing sufficient information for the patient to come to their own decision without duress, and it implies a degree of trust. Usually implicit in this is the understanding that the treatment or procedure being offered is consistent with recognised standard practice.

Without compliance based on mutual understanding, everyday clinical practice could not proceed. For invasive procedures in particular valid consent is essential, implying that sufficient information, including possible alternatives, has been given.

Thus information and choice are involved in the doctor–patient contract. As patients have the right to agree, so they also have the right to refuse. However, they cannot demand a particular treatment if doctors consider it inappropriate. For this reason, the British Medical Association in its Code of Practice on Advance Statements about medical treatment[4] refers to them as advance directives (refusals). However, it would be possible to make a statement to the effect that should one be unable to communicate one's wishes, one would encourage all reasonable steps to be taken to preserve one's life.

This might of course give rise to difficulty in interpretation if the treatment involved scarce or expensive procedures. However, in clinical medicine, each case has to be judged on the basis of its own specific circumstances and decisions made accordingly.

# Background

Advance directives were introduced in the USA following the case of Karen Quinlan. Karen was 21 years of age when in 1975 she developed a permanent vegetative state after taking tranquillisers and alcohol. She was maintained on a respirator with nasogastric feeding. When the Quinlan family realised that there was no prospect of Karen's recovery, they requested that her life support be discontinued. There was no legal precedent for such a decision at that time, and medical opinion was firmly against the proposal. A long legal battle ensued during which the courts involved attempted to determine what Karen's wishes would be in the circumstances then affecting her. In the event, the New Jersey Supreme Court gave permission for Karen to be removed from the respirator. Ironically, as feeding was continued, it was not until 10 years later that Karen died.

Arising from this and subsequent cases, the view developed that it would be much easier to make decisions in similar difficult circumstances if the prior wishes of the patient were known. Subsequently, advance directives have been given statutory recognition in all the states in the USA and in Canadian provinces.

A similar debate took place in the UK in the case of Tony Bland, a young man who developed a permanent vegetative state after sustaining injury in the Hillsborough football stadium disaster. Both his doctors and his parents reached the view that after around two years without any improvement in his condition, artificial feeding should be discontinued. The case eventually reached the House of Lords as the highest court of appeal. The Law Lords sanctioned the with-drawal of feeding, and Tony Bland died around four years after being injured.

In giving judgement, a recommendation was made to the effect that Parliament should consider the issues involved. This led to the creation of the House of Lords Select Committee on Medical Ethics, which published its report in 1994.[5] In this report the term *advance directive* is described as a 'document executed while a patient is competent, concerning his or her preferences about medical treatment in the event of becoming incompetent'. The report commended the development of advance directives, but stopped short of recommending statutory legislation to support them, indicating that doctors are increasingly recognising their ethical obligations towards them, and that in any event case law is moving in the same direction.

The report makes important points concerning the implementation of an advance directive.

- An advance directive may express refusal of any treatment or procedure, which would require the consent of the patient if competent.
- An advance directive should not request any unlawful intervention or omission.
- An advance directive cannot require treatment to be given which the health-care team judge is not clinically appropriate.
- It would be impossible to give advance directives greater legal force without depriving patients of the doctor's professional expertise and the benefit of any new treatments that may have become available since the directive was signed.

This last comment (House of Lords report, paragraph 264) summarises one of the most telling objections to the value of advance directives. Instead of legislation, the report recommended that a code of practice be developed by the colleges and faculties of all the healthcare professions to guide their members. This was taken up by the British Medical Association and resulted in the publication of *Advance Statements About Medical Treatment*.[4] The steering group was widely representative of medicine, nursing and the law. It is to date the most authoritative source of information on the application of advance directives.

In the introduction, the code of practice states unequivocally that the subject of advance directives is quite separate from euthanasia, assisted suicide or allocation of healthcare resources. Such a distinction is clearly not shared universally – witness the support given to advance directives by the Voluntary Euthanasia Society.[6] Academics, too, see the subjects as closely related.[7]

The Law Commission, in its report on mental incapacity,[8] recommended specific statutory recognition of advance directives and included this in its draft bill. However, this has not been taken up by the Government and it now seems unlikely that it will be.

In December 1997 the Lord Chancellor published a consultation document in response to the Law Commission's proposals entitled *Who Decides?*.[9] Following the receipt of responses, the Government's proposals for legislation were published in *Making Decisions*.[10]

The report specifically addresses 'advance statements' and concludes that the guidance contained in case law together with the British Medical Association Code of Practice provide sufficient clarity and flexibility to enable the validity and applicability of advance statements to be decided on a case-by-case basis. Therefore there is no reason for further legislation at present.

However, in the same report the intention to create continuing powers of attorney to include healthcare decisions is outlined, as well as the appointment of managers with similar authority. This may well affect the application of advance directives, as it provides another voice and possible alternative interpretation of the principal's wishes. At the time of writing, no legislation has been included in the Government's programme.

The Human Rights Act 1998 incorporated the articles of the European Convention on Human Rights into UK domestic law as from October 2000. The impact of this is discussed in the sixth edition of *Law and Medical Ethics*[11] (paragraphs 1.63 and 1.64). The authors point out that at the present time the focus of change is at the margins of medical law and the use of judicial review rather than the introduction of major new principles. Somewhat reassuringly, the 'right to life' (Article 2) has been held not to imply a correlative right to die. If anything, however, it seems that the Act will strengthen the recognition of the wishes expressed in an advance directive, rather than alter their interpretation.

In the British Medical Association guidance on withholding and withdrawing life-prolonging medical treatment,[12] the impact of advance refusals is addressed (paragraphs 10.1, 10.2 and 10.3). If these include the refusal of artificial nutrition and hydration and the circumstances envisaged in the directive have occurred, then it must be respected. Also in paragraph 12.1 the request for life-prolonging treatment should be taken into account, but would not be binding.

An important caveat in the British Medical Association's guidance is that an advance refusal of basic care should not preclude the offering of oral nutrition and hydration (paragraphs 10.1 and 3.3).

# Form of advance directive

Although most discussion of advance directives envisages a formal document, signed and witnessed, an oral statement supported by third-party evidence would suffice and have ethical and probably also legal status in appropriate circumstances. However, if an oral statement is referred to, there would be no way of knowing if it was intended to apply to the exact situation that has transpired, or whether the principal has changed their mind and wishes to revoke their declared intention.

That said, for practical purposes it can be assumed that an advance directive is a written document. Since as yet it has no precise statutory recognition, it can take a number of different formats. For example, the Terence Higgins Trust has developed a form with HIV in mind, and the Voluntary Euthanasia Society has also recommended a model form.[6]

The Age Concern publication *Their Rights: Advance Directives and Living Wills Explored*[13] gives detailed information on the creation of an advance directive and model examples. Appendix 11 of that publication includes advice and instruction from an American source which runs to 12 pages and is of such complexity and detail that it might cause all but the most determined to give up the whole idea! However, the publication discusses the ethics, law and practical aspects of advance directives in an accessible manner, and must be the most comprehensive and up-to-date source of information currently available to the public. It can be commended to anyone – professional or lay – who is seeking guidance and information on the subject.

A doctor may be presented with directives that express in detail particular treatments that are applicable to specific disorders, for which consent is expressly withdrawn in advance. These statements may be accompanied by a declaration to the effect that the signatory fears 'degeneration' and indignity more than death. The language used is perforce 'lay' language, and in medical terms it may well lack specificity. Unfortunately, when it comes to enforcing such instructions, it may well be the lack of specificity that leads to problems of interpretation.

However, some advance directives are less ambitious and confine themselves to a values inventory that indicates the patient's likely views if they were to be subject to certain circumstances. Such views could well be helpful to the healthcare team in decision making, especially if coupled with an understanding that some leeway in making those decisions is more likely than not to be in their best interests.

On occasion relatives may offer a simple signed statement which the patient has written in their own words and which may or may not have been witnessed and countersigned. Such a statement has the same status as a formal document, as in the absence of formal statutory recognition it demands respect as indicating the apparent wishes of the patient.

# Legal aspects

An unambiguous and informed advance directive has the same authority as a contemporaneous decision. This common-law right has been confirmed in several legal cases.[14,15] However, as there are no statutory regulations for the creation of an advance directive, how can we be certain that the declaration was based on adequate information and that the signatory was competent at the time? Can we really be certain that the circumstances envisaged are identical to those which have occurred? There are many different factors to be taken into account, of which diagnostic uncertainty is just one.

Nonetheless, the recent judgements referred to above have confirmed the authority of anticipatory refusal. The elements considered necessary derived from those judgements have been summarised by Luttrell as follows.[16]

1　The advance refusal was made by a mentally competent adult.
2　The consequences of the refusal were known to the person when making the refusal.
3　The refusal was intended to apply to the circumstances that have arisen.
4　The decision to refuse treatment was not made under the influence of another party.
5　The refusal has not been subsequently revoked or cancelled.
6　The person making the directive has subsequently become incompetent and incapable of making a decision about their healthcare when such a decision is needed.

These are rigorous standards, but they match the seriousness of the actions that advance directives have power to influence. Stuart Hornett[17] provides a rigorous legal and ethical appraisal of advance directives from a lawyer's viewpoint. He fully recognises the clinical problem that they may create for doctors, and he concludes that there is much to commend the argument that they should inform but not be binding on the doctor. He indicates problems, some of which are quite fundamental, that have yet to be adequately addressed. One such problem is whether a patient who has become incompetent can overrule an advance directive made when he or she was competent.

The British Medical Association Code of Practice draws attention to some of the practical problems concerning the implementation of advance directives in the UK.

1　The question of capacity (paragraph 2.4) is addressed more fully in the British Medical Association and Law Society's joint report on *Assessment of Mental Capacity: guidance for doctors and lawyers*, section 10.6.[18]
2　The problems concerning advance directives are addressed in paragraphs 9.1 and 9.2. These are vital practical issues, as they clearly affect the whole exercise of conceiving, executing and implementing an advance directive. The question of informing the appropriate healthcare team that has responsibility for making decisions concerning the patient is critical.
3　The question of basic care and its definition (paragraph 5.1).
4　Conscientious objection to the implementation of an advance directive (section 13).

In the UK, the British Medical Association Code of Practice is currently the most authoritative and practical guide for healthcare personnel, and should be available in clinical settings where advance directives may be presented for implementation.

# Other issues

The General Medical Council has included advice to doctors on 'advance statements' in its document on consent.[19] This is an important step, as it means that awareness of advance directives and their observance is mandatory.

However, it must be remembered that advance directives originated in North America, where the healthcare system is significantly different from that in the UK (where the majority of patients receive treatment for life-threatening illness within the National Health Service). Constraints on resources may affect clinical practice and limit the choice of procedures that are considered appropriate.

There has been much publicity concerning the cost of care for the elderly, and Government policy is directed towards shifting the financial burden from the State to the individual. This is causing considerable alarm to the elderly, who see their estate being used up in providing for their care instead of being passed to their offspring. The prospect of needing long-term care in a nursing home is viewed with dismay, and without doubt some see the execution of an advance directive as a way of avoiding such an eventuality. It needs to be emphasised that the effect of an advance directive may indeed shorten life in some circumstances, but that it would not necessarily prevent the occurrence of disability due to the gradual effect of chronic conditions. Furthermore, the possibility of coercion by self-interested parties should be kept in mind.

There is little reported evidence of the effectiveness of advance directives in practice. Recent publications suggest a cooling of enthusiasm for them, which may well be due to practical experience of some of the problems to which attention has been drawn.

As there is no statutory registration of advance directives, there is no information available as to how many individuals have executed one. However, experience suggests that at the present time only a very small minority of the public have done so.

If an advance directive is executed by someone who is already suffering from a life-threatening condition, it is more likely to be better informed and thus more precise in its instructions than a document prepared many years earlier when the occurrence of particular illnesses could not have been anticipated and the individual's response to their situation was assumed rather than actually experienced.

# Conclusion

There is no doubt about the ethical basis for advance directives, which derives from recognition of individual autonomy. However, the practical and legal problems surrounding their implementation raise important issues that need to be addressed. If nothing else, the debate on advance directives leads to a discussion of the difficulty of decision making in cases of life-threatening illness. In *Making Decisions*[10] the Government recorded the widely differing views on advance directives, and we can concur with their intention to continue to keep the subject under review in the light of future medical and legal developments.

---

**Key points**

- An advance directive (sometimes known as a living will) is a statement of treatment preferences as an indication of a patient's wishes should his or her capacity for decision making be lost in the future.
- Advance directives have the authority of common-law precedent, but there is no statute law enforcing their format or content.
- For practical purposes an advance directive is normally a written document.
- There are important practical issues concerning the implementation of advance directives which need to be recognised.
- If the Government enacts the proposals contained in *Making Decisions* (although advance directives are to be excluded), the appointment of an attorney or manager for healthcare decisions may affect the way in which such decisions are made in cases of life-threatening illness in incapacitated patients.

---

# References

1  Kutner L (1969) Due process of euthanasia: the Living Will, a proposal. *Indiana Law J.* 44: 539–54.

2  Hope T, Savulescu J and Hendrick J (2003) *Medical Ethics and Law: the core curriculum.* Churchill Livingstone, London.

3  Ms B and an NHS Hospital Trust (2000) EWHC 329 (Fam), (2002) 2 All ER 449, (2002) 65 BMLR 149.

4  British Medical Association (1995) *Advance Statements about Medical Treatment.* British Medical Association, London.

5   House of Lords (1994) *Report of the Select Committee on Medical Ethics*. HMSO, London.

6   Davies J (1997) *Choice in Dying*. Ward Lock, London.

7   McLean S and Britton A (1997) *The Case for Physician-Assisted Suicide*. Harper Collins, London.

8   Law Commission (1995) *Mental Incapacity*. Law Commission Report No. 231. HMSO, London.

9   Lord Chancellor (1997) *Who Decides? Making decisions on behalf of mentally incapacitated adults*. Department of Constitutional Affairs, Lord Chancellor's Office, London.

10  Lord Chancellor (1999) *Making Decisions: the Government's proposals for making decisions on behalf of mentally incapacitated adults*. Department of Constitutional Affairs, Lord Chancellor's Office, London.

11  Mason JK, McCall Smith RA and Laurie GT (2000) *Law and Medical Ethics* (6e). Butterworths, London.

12  British Medical Association (1999) *Withholding or Withdrawing Life-Prolonging Medical Treatment*. British Medical Association, London.

13  Kendrick K and Robinson S (2002) *Their Rights: advance directives and living wills explored*. Age Concern England, London.

14  Re C (adult: refusal of treatment) (1994) 1 WLR 290.

15  Re T (adult: refusal of treatment) (1993) Fam 95.

16  Luttrell S (1996) Living wills do have legal affect provided certain criteria are met. *BMJ*. **313**: 1148.

17  Hornett S (1997) Advance directives: a legal and ethical analysis. In: Keown J (ed.) *Euthanasia Examined*. Cambridge University Press, Cambridge.

18  British Medical Associaiton and Law Society (1995) *Assessment of Mental Capacity: guidance for doctors and lawyers*. British Medical Association, London.

19  General Medical Council (1998) *Seeking Patient Consent: the ethical considerations*. General Medical Council, London.

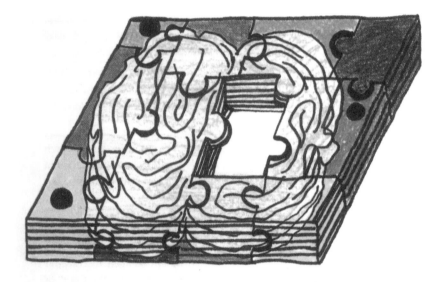

# CHAPTER 9

# Ethical issues in stroke management

*David Sulch and Lalit Kalra*

## Background

Stroke is a major clinical problem. The incidence is 150–250 per 100 000 per year in the UK, equating to a figure of 400–500 per year in an area served by the average district general hospital. Of these patients, 25–30% will die during the first month, and a significant proportion of the survivors will be disabled to a greater or lesser degree. Approximately 15% of survivors will be residing in institutional care one year after the stroke.

The management of stroke patients involves frequent decisions which require careful ethical consideration. In the early stages, decisions must be made against a background of uncertainty regarding the likely outcome. Later, key decisions will be necessary in patients who have been left with severe disability. In addition, many stroke patients are left unable to communicate their wishes with regard to treatment and placement decisions.

## Diagnosis

An accurate diagnosis is essential when formulating decisions about the management of a patient with an apparent stroke. A number of conditions can mimic the clinical syndrome of a stroke, including an intracranial neoplasm, subdural haematoma, intracranial abscess and hypoglycaemia. In addition, the distinction between cerebral infarction and cerebral haemorrhage cannot be accurately made on clinical grounds alone. The key investigation in establishing the diagnosis is brain imaging, via either a computed tomography (CT) scan or a magnetic resonance imaging (MRI) scan. All patients suspected of having a stroke should have a CT scan performed within 48 hours, in accordance with the National Service Framework for Older People.[1] Although these guidelines are clear, there is often an ethical issue with regard to scanning patients who may have a clinically poor prognosis or multiple disorders, where the clinician believes that scanning will not change management or outcome. This may be true in most cases, but there are several instances where investigations do not support initial clinical impressions and reveal an element of reversibility. Refusal to perform such a scan on the grounds of age or disability is unethical, and all patients should have basic investigations except in cases where death is imminent and undertaking investigations is likely to cause distress.

# Prognosis

Accurate early information regarding the prognosis is critical to enable rational decisions to be made about a patient's treatment. To withhold antibiotics from a patient who has a 5% chance of recovery may be ethical – to do the same in a patient with a 50% chance of recovery certainly is not. Unfortunately, decisions not to treat on the basis of a probable poor outcome very often become self-fulfilling prophecies.

In a minority of cases it is clear that the patient has a very poor prognosis. For a patient with an extensive intracerebral bleed and impending coning, or a demented patient with a history of several previous strokes, there is a very poor prognosis. Early decisions to withhold possible life-prolonging measures can be made with confidence in such patients. However, the outlook for most stroke patients is much less clear.

A number of approaches can help to provide prognostic information.

# Adverse prognostic factors

A number of factors that imply a poor prognosis have been identified in research studies. These include the following:

- unconsciousness on admission
- multiple/severe comorbidity
- very advanced age
- cognitive impairment
- pre-existing dependence.

Of these, a low level of consciousness on admission is the most secure indication of a poor prognosis.

# Subtype

The Bamford classification (as used in the Oxfordshire Community Stroke Project[2]) subdivides strokes into four groups as follows:

1   *lacunar* – pure motor, pure sensory, sensorimotor or ataxic hemiplegia
2   *total anterior circulation (TACS)* – higher cortical dysfunction (dysphasia or visuospatial neglect), homonymous hemianopia and hemiplegia and/or sensory deficit involving at least two of face, arm and leg
3   *partial anterior circulation (PACS)* – two of the three components of TACS, higher dysfunction alone or motor/sensory deficit more restricted than those classified as lacunar events
4   *posterior circulation (POCS)* – homonymous hemianopia alone, crossed cranial nerve palsies (e.g. Weber's syndrome), cerebellar syndrome without long tract signs, bilateral motor/sensory deficit.

The prognosis for these subtypes is very different. More than 50% of patients with TACS are dead one year after their stroke, and the majority of those who survive a TACS will remain dependent on care to a greater or lesser degree. In contrast, death following a lacunar event is uncommon (less than 10% of cases at one year), and the majority of these patients will regain full independence.

# Aetiology

Intracerebral haemorrhage confers a worse prognosis than cerebral infarction. The mortality at one month following a bleed approaches 50%, compared with 15% for infarction.[3]

# Scoring scales

A number of scores have proved accurate in assessing the prognosis when applied between two and four weeks after a stroke. Recent work suggests that the National Institute of Health Stroke Scale (NIHSS) may confer an accurate probability of recovery if used in the first week (*see* Figure 9.1).[4] A score higher than 16 implies a poor prognosis, while one below 6 implies a good prognosis.

   There are therefore a number of factors which can be taken into account when attempting to provide a patient and their family with accurate information about the likelihood of recovery. An accurate estimate of a patient's chances of improvement provides a framework to aid in decision making. However, it must be remembered that the presentation in an individual patient is key, and that patients who at face value would appear to have a poor prognosis may do surprisingly well.

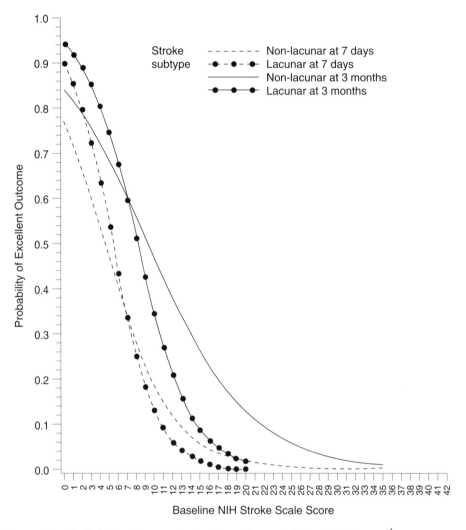

**Figure 9.1**   Probability of an excellent outcome from stroke by NIHSS score.[4]

---

**Case 1**

A previously well 69-year-old man was admitted with a dense left hemiplegia. He was semi-conscious with a Glasgow Coma Score (GCS) of 9. A CT
scan showed a large basal ganglia bleed with mass effect. Despite the bleed
and the low GCS, it was felt that he might do well once the haematoma had
resolved. Aggressive supportive treatment including nasogastric feeding
and antibiotics were used. His GCS rose to 15 three weeks after admission,

and after rehabilitation he was discharged home, requiring only a small amount of help with personal care.

# Drug treatment

The issue of thrombolysis in the early management of stroke patients remains controversial. A meta-analysis of all studies demonstrates benefit if recombinant tissue plasminogen activator (r-tPA) is administered within three hours to an appropriate group of patients.[5] Clinicians in some centres in the world would regard non-administration of thrombolysis to a suitable patient as unethical. However, in the UK thrombolysis has only recently been licensed for stroke patients, and a majority view suggests that UK clinicians require further training before the general use of thrombolysis can be implemented routinely in clinical practice. Their previous concerns about the security of the evidence, particularly since the majority of the benefit seen in the meta-analysis derives from one study (the NINDS trial[6]), have now been resolved and further highlight the value of thrombolysis. A recent Cochrane meta-analysis also supports a six-hour time window, highlighting an even greater role for thrombolytic therapy. Several large multicentre trials, such as the IST-III and ECASS-III, are currently under way to evaluate whether extending the time window and thrombolysis in non-specialist centres are feasible and effective. Until this has been ascertained, thrombolysis should be restricted to larger specialised centres with experience in the technique, because of the high risk of haemorrhage.

# Nutrition and hydration

Approximately 45% of stroke patients will have some degree of dysphagia and associated aspiration immediately after their stroke. This will resolve in over 90% of cases during the next three months. Many of these patients will be able to take a soft diet, but some will have a severe degree of dysphagia that precludes oral feeding, and will require an alternative route to be found.

The provision of nutrition and hydration has been regarded as different to the provision of medical treatments. The law regards nutrition and hydration as a basic human right. However, the issue is clouded because both of the means used to provide nutrition and hydration in dysphasic stroke patients (nasogastric tubes and intravenous cannulae) fall under the heading of medical interventions. Thus it can be argued that such treatments (as with any medical treatment) can be provided or withheld at the discretion of the treating medical team.

In practice, virtually no clinician would withhold hydration from a dysphasic stroke patient. However, decisions concerning nutrition are perceived as more complex, because the means used to provide nutrition (nasogastric tubes) are deemed more uncomfortable (and thus less acceptable) than the means used to provide hydration. To complicate matters further, there remains a dearth of high-quality research evidence to guide decisions concerning nutrition (particularly the timing of initiation of enteral feeding), although a major multicentre trial (the FOOD study) is currently in progress. The evidence currently available (from a non-randomised study) suggests that nutrition in the first 72 hours may improve the prognosis.

In our view, withholding nutrition from a stroke patient in the early stages is unethical unless the prognosis is clearly hopeless. Our practice is to commence nasogastric feeding on the day after admission. Whether nasogastric feeding is the route of choice remains undetermined. Very often patients pull out nasogastric tubes with their good hand, increasing the probability of complications associated with repeated tube insertion. There are also ethical issues surrounding the use of restraint to prevent such patients from dislodging nasogastric tubes. Gastrostomy tubes provide a more secure route for feeding, as well as a more reliable supply of nutrition. However, at present there is no evidence to support the immediate use of gastrostomy tubes, and their insertion requires a surgical procedure and exposes the patient to potential complications.

# Withdrawal of feeding

Withdrawal of nutrition at a later date in a patient who has not improved and who remains very disabled may be an appropriate action. If one regards nutrition via tube feeding as a medical intervention, then according to the medical model, if the indication for such an intervention no longer exists, that intervention can be withdrawn. Certainly decisions concerning the withdrawal of life-prolonging interventions can be made without legal recourse, and indeed are made on a daily basis in intensive-care units across the country. This is of course a potentially emotive subject, but discussions of this nature can be made much easier if there is appropriate counselling of the relatives before feeding is commenced. It may remain very difficult to withdraw such nutrition in a conscious patient because of fears about the symptomatic effects of lack of nutrition, and in practice nutrition is often continued more as a palliative intervention, long after there is any hope of a meaningful recovery.

# Chest infection and antibiotics

The high incidence of dysphagia coupled with other factors, such as reduced mobility, under-nutrition and exposure to hospital pathogens, means that chest infection (and more specifically pneumonia) is a common problem in patients with acute stroke. In a severely disabled stroke patient, clinicians are often faced with the difficult decision of whether to treat such an infection, or whether it is kinder to withhold medication and allow nature to take its course. The latter decision is difficult to support in the early stages of stroke treatment, in view of the doubts discussed earlier about the accuracy of prognostic decisions in the early stages. One may also note that the administration of intravenous antibiotics is acceptable and generally not distressing to the patient and their relatives, even allowing for the potential side-effects of such agents. Thus it is common practice (and ethically sound) to treat all such infections in the early stages of stroke management. The situation may be very different if the same patient with the same severe degree of disability develops pneumonia three months later. By this stage, the lack of potential for further recovery is clear and a decision to withhold treatment is ethically and morally supportable.

# Resuscitation orders

Much controversy exists over the rationale behind the allocation of 'do not attempt resuscitation' (DNAR) orders. The tendency in stroke cases (more than in most other conditions that represent acute medicine) is for a high proportion of patients admitted with this condition to be allocated a DNAR order. This is often done without consultation with the patient or their relatives.

Medically there are sound reasons why DNAR orders may be appropriate in stroke patients, even in the acute setting. The majority of patients who suffer a cardiac arrest in hospital, but who are successfully resuscitated and survive to discharge, are those with reversible acute cardiac conditions (e.g. myocardial infarction). One study suggests that stroke patients who undergo cardiopulmonary resuscitation (CPR) have a 6% chance of survival to discharge, compared with 20% for the general hospital population.[7] Concern has also been raised about the detrimental effects of the resuscitation process on cerebral perfusion in a patient who is already suffering a degree of brain injury. It is feared that a stroke patient who survives a resuscitation effort will be left with a more severe degree of brain injury and thus greater disability.

However, studies of CPR outcome in hospital have often excluded large numbers of stroke patients because of the frequency with which they are allocated DNAR orders, and may not provide a true picture of the potential for survival among such patients. It must also be remembered that stroke patients often have coexistent ischaemic heart disease, which has the potential to cause transient, treatable arrhythmia (e.g. ventricular fibrillation). Many stroke patients, particularly those with lacunar infarcts, have a very good prognosis, and issuing such a patient with a DNAR order solely because they have had a stroke is unlikely to be defensible.

Should one consult the patient? It is generally accepted that it is good practice to involve the patient in such decisions. Resuscitation is after all a medical intervention, and ethically and legally the patient has a right to accept or reject any medical interventions they are offered. Indeed, research studies strongly suggest that patients feel that such decisions are theirs alone to make. Equally, however, as with any medical intervention, it is the clinician's responsibility to make the final decision as to whether such an intervention is appropriate for any individual patient. Until recently it was acceptable for the doctor not to involve the patient in the decision if CPR was likely to be futile or if discussion of the issue was deemed likely to be harmful (i.e. to cause anxiety or distress). However, the new guidelines reject the use of the term 'futility' in considering DNAR decisions. The guidance suggests that doctors should consider the prospects for restoration of pulse and respiration and then whether this would be of benefit for the patient, and it advises them to recognise the fact that a competent person can refuse a DNAR order and doctors must respect this decision.

The situation is more difficult when the patient is unable either to communicate their wishes or to understand the issue. Attempts to predict the patient's wishes in this situation are generally inaccurate – studies suggest that clinicians underestimate patients' desire to undergo CPR.[8] It is generally suggested that the relatives should be consulted in this situation (although they tend to overestimate a patient's desire to undergo CPR). Certainly the clinician has a duty to discuss and inform the patient and their advocate of possible outcomes and variables which may affect the prognosis. However, it should again be stressed that this decision is ultimately a medical decision, and the clinician who acts in the patient's best interests should not be criticised. Indeed, clinicians have a moral responsibility to state their view of the appropriateness of a resuscitation decision, and must not leave the responsibility for this decision to the family alone.

---

**Case 2**

A 58-year-old man suffered a large intracerebral bleed, with a resulting dense hemiplegia, hemianopia and dysphasia. Three months after his stroke he was transferred to another hospital for further management. No clear decision regarding resuscitation status had been made at the first hospital. A series of difficult interviews were held with the patient's family. The medical staff made clear their view that a DNAR order should be issued. The family were opposed to this, but after much debate admitted that they would never initiate a DNAR order because they felt that this would tantamount to killing their relative. After many discussions, they eventually agreed with the medical viewpoint, and the order was issued.

Finally, it must be understood that a decision not to resuscitate is not the same as a decision not to treat, and that issues concerning the administration of anti-biotics, etc. are quite separate.

# Placement

A common problem in the later stages of stroke treatment concerns issues about discharge. Two basic rules are unavoidable. The patient should be discharged to where they wish to go if at all possible, and although this may not always be possible, no patient should be forcibly discharged to somewhere they do not wish to go. The patient's right to self-determination as enshrined in law requires these conditions to be met.

Problems arise in those patients who refuse to accept the danger of returning to an unsuitable environment. The law is quite clear about this situation – a mentally competent adult has the right to do what they wish, and the clinician must accede to their wishes. In cases of mental incompetence or lack of insight, a psychiatrist may certify that a patient is unable to understand the issues being considered, and placement in what the multi-disciplinary team regard as the appropriate environment can then be facilitated. Often this can be achieved with careful liaison with the patient's family and other interested parties, without recourse to the courts. However, if there is continuing difficulty, it may be necessary to apply for a guardianship order under Section 7 of the Mental Health Act 1983. This permits the placement of the individual in a safe environment even against their expressed wishes. Patients who are unable to express their wishes must be managed in accordance with their 'best interests', although care needs to be taken to try to enable such patients to indicate their views as much as possible.

---

**Case 3**

A disabled 68-year-old stroke survivor was readmitted to hospital with a urinary tract infection. He was severely dysphasic, and previous assessment had indicated that he was inconsistent with regard to his 'yes' and 'no' responses. He had been living with his partner of ten years, but his son demanded that the patient should return to live with him, as he did not believe that the partner was caring for his father appropriately. A further speech therapy opinion was requested. The therapist saw the patient together with a psychiatrist, and established that the patient was now consistent in his 'yes' and 'no' responses. The patient expressed a wish to return to his partner.

---

# Dysphasia

Many stroke patients are left unable to express their views about their treatment by virtue of the development of dysphasia as a complication of their stroke. As in the above example, skilled and patient assessment by a speech and language therapist may establish that the patient can communicate their wishes in some way. In those who cannot do so, the wishes of the family should clearly be considered. Legally, however, no adult can either give or withhold consent for any procedure on behalf of another adult. There is no mechanism in English law by which such decision making can be made by a proxy. For example, an enduring power of attorney merely gives a relative control over the patient's financial matters, and provides them with no power to make decisions about healthcare. Thus the final responsibility for healthcare decisions rests with the multi-disciplinary team, who should act in accordance with the patient's best interests at all times (this may include authorising surgical procedures such as gastrostomy tube insertion).

# Driving after stroke

Legally, patients who have suffered a stroke or transient ischaemic attack should not drive for a month after the event. The patient should be advised to inform the DVLA and their insurance company. After a month, patients may resume driving if this is deemed safe by their clinician. In cases of doubt, an assessment at a Driver Assessment Unit may provide confirmation of a patient's degree of fitness to drive.

Some manifestations of stroke (e.g. homonymous hemianopia) disqualify the patient from driving. The clinician is negligent if they do not inform the patient of this fact, and can be held legally liable should an accident ensue. If a patient who is unfit to drive is known to be continuing to drive and will not inform the DVLA, the clinician can break confidentiality and inform the DVLA him- or herself. In these circumstances the clinician's responsibility to society outweighs their responsibility to maintain confidentiality.

**Key points**

- Only in a minority of stroke patients is it possible to state that their prognosis is virtually hopeless within the first few days.
- All patients other than those with no chance of recovery should receive nutrition and hydration, and should have brain imaging performed.

- Withdrawal of treatment may be justified in a patient in whom a poor prognosis has become clearer with the passage of time.
- Other potentially life-saving treatments (e.g. antibiotics) should not be withheld while the prognosis is uncertain.
- It is acceptable to issue a DNAR order while continuing all other treatments.
- It is unacceptable to issue a DNAR order to a patient solely because they have had a stroke.
- The clinician is ethically and legally justified in deciding treatments that are in the patient's best interests for those who cannot express their wishes.
- Communication with patients and relatives at all stages is the best way to ensure acceptability of decisions.

# References

1  Department of Health (2001) *National Service Framework for Older People*; www.doh.gov. uk/nsf/olderpeople.htm

2  Bamford J, Sandercock P, Dennis M, Burn J and Warlow C (1991) Classification and natural history of clinically identifiable subtypes of cerebral infarction. *Lancet.* **337**: 1521–6.

3  Dennis M, Burn J, Sandercock P, Bamford J, Wade D and Warlow C (1993) Long-term survival after first-ever stroke: the Oxfordshire Community Stroke Project. *Stroke.* **24**: 1084–9.

4  Adams H, Davis P, Leira E *et al.* (1999) Baseline NIH Stroke Scale score strongly predicts outcome after stroke: a report of the Trial of Org 10172 in Acute Stroke Treatment (TOAST). *Neurology.* **53**: 126–31.

5  Wardlaw JM, del Zoppo G, Yamaguchi T and Berge E (2003) Thrombolysis for acute ischaemic stroke (Cochrane Review). In: *Cochrane Library. Issue 3*. Update Software, Oxford.

6  Kwiatkowski T, Libman R, Frankel M *et al.* (1999) Effects of tissue plasminogen activator for acute ischaemic stroke at 1 year. *NEJM.* **340**: 1781–7.

7  de Vos R, Koster R, De Haan R *et al.* (1999) In-hospital cardiopulmonary resuscitation: pre-arrest morbidity and outcome. *Arch Intern Med.* **159**: 845–50.

8  Uhlmann R, Pearlman R and Cain K (1988) Physicians' and spouses' predictions of elderly patients' resuscitation preferences. *J Gerontol.* **43**: 115–21.

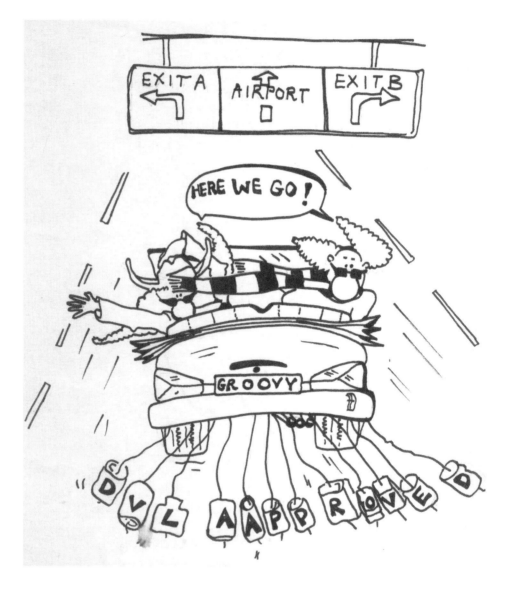

# CHAPTER 10

# Ethics of driving assessment in dementia: care, competence and communication

## *David Robinson and Desmond O'Neill*

## Background

'We are bringing you to Dr O'Neill so that he can put you in a nursing home' would be a poor advertisement for a prospective patient with age-related disease about to attend a geriatric medicine clinic. The reasons for the unease generated by this phrase for both patients and practitioners are a useful guide to some of the issues related to ethics and driving. Both groups would be much happier with a formula along the lines of 'We are bringing you to Dr O'Neill to maximise your chances of staying at home. Of course, at some stage you may no longer be able to manage at home, and we may need to consider other options in the future.'

So what is the difference? The second formula:

- puts the needs and wishes of the patient to the fore, rather than those of the carer or of society
- promotes the concept of geriatric medicine as enabling rather than disabling
- recognises a style of practice consistent with World Health Organization (WHO)[1] and United Nations (UN)[2] guidelines which promotes due attention to prevention, health gain, health maintenance and palliation
- recognises the role of geriatric medicine in changing a societal mind-set towards disabling conditions of later life. Prior to the pioneering work of Marjorie Warren, the response of society was a prosthetic one, reinforcing disability by premature admission to residential care. The key advance of geriatric medicine was to bring a diagnostic and therapeutic emphasis to the care of older people.

The contextual setting of the ethics of driving often seems to neglect the simple principles of care, competence and communication outlined above – 'care' in the sense of the appropriate focus of the practitioner–patient interaction, 'competence' in the sense of knowing not only the literature of assessment and remediation but also the extent of societal ageism, and 'communication' in the sense of understanding the skills needed to move from a primary focus on health gain to one of palliation. The primary ethos still appears to be 'We are bringing you to Dr O'Neill so that he can stop your driving' rather than 'We are bringing you to Dr O'Neill to maximise your chances of maintaining your mobility and transportation. Of course, at some stage you may no longer be able to drive, and we may need to consider other options in the future.' The literature in this area is a gloomy testament to the under-developed nature of the debate. The vast majority of the papers on Medline still focus on who should not drive, rather than considering the health implications of inadequate access to transport.

# Public health ethics

The mis-emphasis probably arises from the processing of data by public health specialists whose primary role is the interpretation of accident analysis. An ethical imperative for such public health professionals is to become aware of the due proportionality of mobility and safety, and the importance of maintaining this balance in later life. This raises further issues with regard to how to ensure an input of gerontological training for public health professionals.

The challenge to geriatricians and gerontologists in relation to age-related disease and driving is to realign the context of mobility and risk. Some progress has already been made in this regard – the major impact of age-related disease is to curtail mobility.[3] A more measured sense of perspective has allowed a previous emphasis on risk to be reviewed – it is clear that older drivers are one of the safest groups of drivers on the road. A recent Organisation for Economic Co-operation and Development (OECD) report,[4] entitled *Ageing and Transport*, has re-emphasised that the main public health concerns of ageing and driving are first reduced mobility and secondly the hazard of increased frailty in an automotive and traffic environment that is not tailored to the needs of older people. Although older people as a group are the safest category of drivers on the road, the OECD pointed out the need for wider diffusion of assessment routines for clinicians dealing with drivers with known age-related disease.

# Driving: a right and a privilege

Certain publications on driving assert that the possession of a driving licence is a privilege, but in reality it is probably both a right and a privilege. All of our societies place a higher premium on mobility than on safety. If safety were the first priority, then the speed limit would be 20 miles per hour and car engines would be fitted with governors to prevent them exceeding this speed. The right to drive carries an implicit understanding of bearing a risk that is within certain societal norms. At all levels, older drivers as a group bear a risk that is low. A false argument is sometimes presented that their accident rate per mile travelled is high. This is false for two reasons. First, because they drive a lower mileage, their annual risk remains low. Secondly, low mileage is intrinsically risky. If older and younger drivers are controlled for low mileage, their apparent increased risk disappears.[5]

These positive aspects of ageing are often under-appreciated, and the literature on ageing and mobility could benefit from a greater emphasis on the beneficial aspects of ageing. These include wisdom, strategic thinking and less risk taking. Even within the small proportion of crashes caused by drivers in this age group, the contribution of chronic disease to the crash risk is modest.[6] The safety record of older drivers in the face of these odds points to superior strategic and tactical skills. If skills were more widely applied, these qualities could enhance mobility and safety for all age groups.

# Ethical hazards in clinical settings

The ethical risks to practitioners in clinical practice are failure to consider driving as a part of their patient's functional status, a tendency to police rather than to enable, failure to refer appropriately for competence assessment, and inappropriate disclosure of information. The most striking example of failure to consider driving as a health-related issue comes from a study at a syncope clinic where referring physicians failed to alert many drivers (including lorry drivers!) to stop driving until assessment and treatment were concluded.[7] It is likely that this agnosia is widespread among the profession, but it will probably wane with time.

Against this background it is important to remember the primary duties and ethical responsibilities of the physician. First, to do no harm implies avoiding the damage to lifestyle, self-esteem and subsequently health that restrictions on driving may incur. For this reason we prefer to emphasise the empowering role of the physician – there is already much emphasis in the literature on limiting a patient's ability to drive. It is a physician's duty to promote the well-being of his patient, and it is important to remind ourselves and our patients that our role should be to enable patients to fulfil their potential, rather than to restrict it. Respecting patients' autonomy should enable us to allow patients to accept their own risk, but all too often they are not given this choice.

There has been a modest but significant increase in the literature on disease and driving. Some of this is original research and some represents a synthesis of prevailing wisdom. In many areas, physicians have more information than they did ten years ago. For example, with implantable cardiac defibrillators we know that the risk of crashes due to the defibrillator is low,[8] and we can predict those most at risk for syncope.[9] For cataracts, we know that older drivers with cataract experience a restriction in their driving mobility and a decrease in their safety on the road.[10] We also know that surgical intervention can benefit older patients in terms of subjectively improved visual function and distance estimation while driving.[11] For arthritis, we know not only that doctors fail to enquire about the impact of arthritis on mobility,[12] but also that a rehabilitative intervention programme can improve driving ease.[13] For diabetes, we have increasing evidence that the condition on its own has little or no effect on crash risk among older drivers without a history of crashes.

# Assessment

The assessment of patients' driving ability therefore requires certain minimum standards in order to assess fairly both ability to drive and risk to others. This involves remaining up to date with best practice, being aware of local legislation, and remaining cognizant of the massive impact that we have on a person's lifestyle. The competence required is that patients will have the most accurate assessment possible of their driving abilities. Although schemata exist for the preliminary work in this area for physicians in primary care (e.g. the UK,[14] Australia,[15] Canada,[16] and the USA[17]) and the American Medical Association have produced a physician's guide to assessing and counselling older drivers and have developed a training of trainers course based on this guide to educate physicians on issues of older driver safety and to train them on assessing and counselling medical fitness to drive. Details of these courses will be available on www.ama-assn.org from spring 2004.

Just as not all chest pains arise from pulmonary emboli, clinicians need to have access to appropriate specialist expertise and technology to exclude the diagnosis in such cases. So, too, general physicians may need to invoke the assistance of a driving specialist centre, the components of which are medicine, occupational therapy, sometimes neuropsychology, and specialist driving assessors. A first effort may be made with a suitably trained occupational therapist – this profession is notable for upskilling in driving assessment in Australia, Canada and the USA. If this assessment is inconclusive, an on-road assessment is advisable. In the UK, such assessments are available from the Forum group of driver assessment centres. In the USA, the Association of Driver Rehabilitation Specialists (ADED; www.aded.net) can provide a list of suitably qualified driving assessors. It is important to emphasise to the patient that this test is not the driving test used for learner drivers, but rather it is an assessment designed to gain insight into the capabilities and difficulties of the driver.

# Therapeutic management and risk assessment

It is the placing of driving issues in an appropriate therapeutic context that is perhaps the most important task – non-clinician bioethicists thrive on the artificial heightening of potential conflict inherent in such situations. Rather than focusing on the difficult issue of patients who present late with impaired driving ability and insight, we need to recognise that the assessment of dementia provides the potential for a range of interventions, one of the most important of which is the establishment of a framework for advance planning in a progressive disease. Just as this is commonly recognised for such practical matters as enduring power of attorney in many jurisdictions, so too we need to start a process which encompasses an assessment and a commitment to maximising mobility, but also a process of awareness raising for the patient and their carers that the progression of the disease will inevitably result in a loss of driving capacity. This latter component has been termed a Ulysses contract (after the hero who made his crew tie him to the mast of the ship on the condition that they did not heed his entreaties to be released when seduced by the song of the sirens).[18] Developing this process incorporates some new stances in dementia care, in particular disclosure of the diagnosis in at least general terms – the patient who drives needs to be told that they have a memory problem that is likely to progress and hamper their driving abilities. In general, carers are fearful of diagnosis disclosure but older people seem to want to be told if they have this illness. There is also evidence that such a process may facilitate driver cessation, by enhancing a therapeutic dimension to disease diagnosis and advance planning.[19] It forms the basis of a useful patient and carer brochure from the Hartford Foundation, which is also available online.[20]

The commitment to maximising mobility must focus first on as accurate an assessment of the patient's driving abilities as possible, and secondly on exploring and planning alternative options for a future when driving is no longer possible. It is the promise of an attempt to maximise mobility that is the key to this transaction. If this is not a central component, we are faced with a dual ethical hazard. In the first instance, the therapeutic role of medicine is subjugated to an approach which inverts the standard mobility/safety ratio to which we are all entitled. A further concern is that people with dementia may avoid assessment of the illness early in its course out of fear of unreasonable restriction of their mobility. As early diagnosis, treatment and management are considered to be desirable, this would be an unwelcome development.

The very act of highlighting the potential for compromised driving ability may have a therapeutic benefit, promoting increased vigilance on the part of the patient and carers about the fact that their social contract for driving privileges is not the same as that of the general public. Some support is given to this concept by the success of restricted licensing for people with medical illnesses in the state of Utah.[21] Although some of the effect might be due to the restrictions (avoidance of motorways and night-time driving), it is also possible that the very act of labelling these drivers may heighten their self-awareness.

The ethical component of risk is the onus on the physician to ensure that this has been assessed in the most accurate and professional manner possible. The greatest risk is to fail to refer the patient on for full assessment, perhaps on the basis that such expertise is geographically distant. Bear in mind that we would not let this deter us from arranging specialist neuroradiology for a suspected subdural haematoma or a ventilation/perfusion scan for a possible pulmonary embolus. We should apply similar criteria to the need for specialised assessments for impaired older drivers, particularly in view of the potential risk to other road users.

# Disclosure and confidentiality

In general, the welfarist role of the physician extends to reminding the patient that most insurance companies require disclosure by the driver of 'illnesses relevant to driving' when they arise. Two issues arise. First, the medical advisers of the insurance companies may not make calculations of insurance rates (or continued insurance) on the basis of reason and evidence, but rather on ageist grounds and prejudice against disability. We may be unwittingly exposing the patient to this prejudice. The answer to this lies in continued advocacy by professional groups at a societal level as well as support by the physician in individual cases if the assessment supports preserved driving skills. A second issue is whether it is sufficient to recommend disclosure to someone who will not remember this advice. However, the physician's role is primarily to ensure safe mobility, and in general it is reasonable to assume that removal of insurance cover is a secondary matter in such cases. It is reasonable to share the disclosure information with the carers.

The actual process of breaking confidentiality in the event of evidence of hazard to other members of the public is almost universally supported by most codes of medical practice. However, the question of to whom this should be reported poses some ethical challenges. The traditional route of reporting to driver licensing authorities (Division of Motor Vehicles [DMV] in the USA, and DVLA in the UK) may have relatively little benefit, as removal of a driving licence is likely to have little impact on many drivers whose insight into deteriorating driving skills is poor. It is important that this disclosure has some likelihood of impact and results in the least traumatic removal of the compromised older driver from the road. In such instances, the family may be able to intervene in terms of disabling the car and providing alternative modes of transport. In our own experience, we rarely have to invoke official intervention, but find that a personal communication with a senior police officer in the patient's locality may result in a sensitive visit to the patient and cessation of driving.

Mandatory reporting presents a different ethical challenge. It is unlikely that it is of significant benefit, and unless such benefit can be shown in future studies from mandatory reporting, the profession should resist the introduction of such schemes and fight against the maintenance of established schemes. For individual practitioners in jurisdictions where such regulations exist, a twin-track approach is probably necessary, involving professional advocacy with law makers, and a considered approach as to whether disclosure is in the patient's best interests on a case-by-case basis. If the physician is confident that the state or province has a mechanism for fair assessment and an enlightened approach to maintaining mobility, compliance is not difficult. If the assessment is cursory and aimed at unduly restricting mobility, physicians may be faced with a problem that is recognised with other laws which may put patients' welfare at risk, and where professional obligations may require non-compliance with an unfair law.

# Conclusion

The inclusion of driver assessment in clinical practice represents a new departure for the disciplines of applied ethics and ageing studies. It presents both challenges and opportunities, and involves not only clinicians but also public health professionals in ensuring that our practice represents a judicious balance between beneficence and non-maleficence, while at the same time keeping a firm perspective on the major issue, which is impaired mobility. The critical elements of care, competence and communication are the fundamentals of clinical practice which help to illuminate and clarify this equilibrium.

---

**Legal points**

- In most countries, the legal obligation to disclose medical conditions that may impair driving lies with the driver.
- Professional codes of conduct usually allow for breaking of medical confidentiality in the case of considered assessments of dangerous driving when such drivers will not cease driving.
- Courts in the UK have considered that doctors are bound to advise patients on conditions which may impair safe driving.[22]

# References

1 World Health Organization (2002) *Active Ageing: a policy framework*. World Health Organization, Geneva.

2 United Nations (2002) *Report of the Second World Assembly on Ageing*. United Nations, New York.

3 Millar WJ (1999) Older drivers – a complex public health issue. *Health Rep*. **11**: 59–71.

4 Organisation for Economic Co-operation and Development (2001) *Ageing and Transport: mobility needs and safety issues*. Organisation for Economic Co-operation and Development, Paris.

5 Hakamies-Blomqvist L, Ukkonen T and O'Neill D (2002) Driver ageing does not cause higher accident rates per mile. *Transport Res Part F, Traffic Psychol Behav*. **5**: 271–4.

6 McGwin G Jr, Sims RV, Pulley L and Roseman JM (2000) Relations among chronic medical conditions, medications and automobile crashes in the elderly: a population-based case–control study. *Am J Epidemiol*. **152**: 424–31.

7 MacMahon M, O'Neill D and Kenny RA (1996) Syncope: driving advice is frequently overlooked. *Postgrad Med J*. **72**: 561–3.

8 Trappe HJ, Wenzlaff P and Grellman G (1998) Should patients with implantable cardioverter–defibrillators be allowed to drive? Observations in 291 patients from a single center over an 11-year period. *J Cardiovasc Electrophysiol*. **2**: 93–201.

9 Bansch D, Brunn J, Castrucci M *et al*. (1998) Syncope in patients with an implantable cardioverter–defibrillator: incidence, prediction and implications for driving restrictions. *J Am Coll Cardiol*. **31**: 608–15.

10 Owsley C, Stalvey B, Wells J and Sloane ME (1999) Older drivers and cataract: driving habits and crash risk. *J Gerontol A Biol Sci Med Sci*. **54**: M203–11.

11 Monestam E and Wachtmeister L (1997) Impact of cataract surgery on car driving: a population-based study in Sweden. *Br J Ophthalmol*. **81**: 16–22.

12 Thevenon A, Grimbert P, Dudenko P, Heuline A and Delcambre B (1989) Polarthrite rhumatoïde et conduite automobile. *Rev Rhum Mal Osteoartic*. **56**: 101–3.

13 Jones JG, McCann J and Lassere MN (1991) Driving and arthritis. *Br J Rheumatol*. **30**: 361–4.

14 Driver and Vehicle Licensing Agency (DVLA) (2000) *At a Glance*. DVLA, Swansea.

15 Austroads (2001) *Assessing Fitness to Drive*. Austroads, Haymarket, NSW.

16 Canadian Medical Association (2000) *Determining Medical Fitness to Drive* (6e). Canadian Medical Association, Ottawa.

17 American Medical Association (2003) *Assessing Fitness to Drive in Older People*. American Medical Association, Chicago.

18 Howe E (2000) Improving treatments for patients who are elderly and have dementia. *J Clin Ethics*. **11**: 291–303.

19  Bahro M, Silber E, Box P and Sunderland T (1995) Giving up driving in Alzheimer's disease – an integrative therapeutic approach. *Int J Geriatr Psychiatry.* **10**: 871–4.

20  Hartford Foundation (2000) *At the Crossroads: a guide to Alzheimer's disease, dementia and driving.* Hartford Foundation, Hartford, CT.

21  Vernon DD, Diller EM, Cook LJ, Reading JC, Suruda AJ and Dean JM (2002) Evaluating the crash and citation rates of Utah drivers licensed with medical conditions, 1992–1996. *Accid Anal Prev.* **34**: 237–46.

22  Medical Defence Union (1999) Driving licence revoked. *J MDU.* **15**: 18.

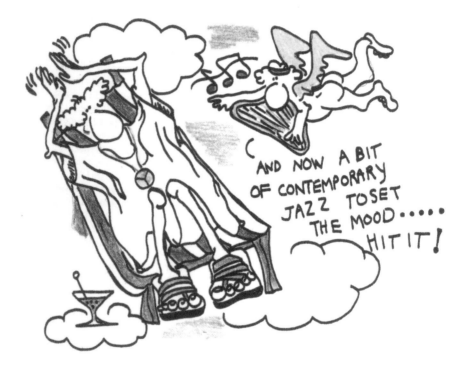

# CHAPTER 11

# Achieving a good death

## Nick Coni and Catherine McAdam

## Introduction

There are 50 000 to 100 000 'sudden' deaths in the UK each year due to natural causes, the usual underlying pathologies being coronary artery disease, massive stroke and pulmonary embolism. Of the expected deaths many are foreseeable, with heart disease, cancer, stroke and respiratory disease being the major killers. A mercifully rapid final illness after enjoyment of an active life almost to the end is highly desirable, but in old age this is often not the outcome.

Traditionally, the term 'euthanasia', derived from the Greek words *eu* and *thanatos*, has simply meant 'a good death', but today it refers to the ending of life of a person who is suffering from advanced incurable illness, for his or her benefit, by another. What constitutes a 'good death'? The answer is three factors – the time to die, the place and the manner of death.

## The time to die

The right time to die is when the body can no longer sustain viable life, and this is usually in old age, which is just as well since almost 80% of deaths in the UK occur in people over 65 years.

## The place to die

Most people, if asked, feel that they would prefer to die in their own homes, but the majority of us in the event die in institutions. Over half (54%) of all deaths occur in NHS hospitals, 13% in private hospitals, residential care homes and nursing homes, and 4% in hospices. The remaining 29% occur in private households or elsewhere, such as in public places. To a varying extent, the doctor may have some influence over both where and how his or her patient dies.

# The way to die

There are many aspects of how we die, and here the doctor may have an important role.

Three principles proposed by Jeffery and Millard[1] provide the doctor with tools to solve moral dilemmas at the end of life. These are as follows.

1   *Treatment of patients must reflect the inherent dignity of every person irrespective of age, debility, dependence, race, colour or creed.* The basis of the ancient Hippocratic oath is respect for the person as an individual in all aspects of medical and nursing management, including the period when withdrawal of treatment is being considered. The value of the person does not depend on whether treatment is useful or not.
2   *Actions taken must reflect the needs of the patient where he or she is.* Doctors' actions should not only display the highest standards of professional behaviour, but should also consider perceived burdens and benefits to the patient, their family, staff, the hospital and the community.
3   *Decisions taken must value the person and accept human mortality.* Although it is the doctor's duty to do no harm, it is not his or her duty to preserve life at all costs. When a medical treatment or intervention is no longer appropriate to sustain life, or the means used to sustain life are out of proportion to the life achieved, death should be accepted and allowed to take its course.

# Dilemmas faced by doctors when dealing with death

## Should the doctor tell or not tell?

The current practice is to adopt a policy of honesty and to share information with the patient – in theory, at least. In fact, few of us really practise what we preach. We may tell the patient of our suspicion that there is something sinister going on until that suspicion has been confirmed. Even then we may put something of a gloss on it in order not to destroy all hope. However, although patients have a right to know, perhaps they also have a right *not* to know. We are all familiar with patients who seem to desist pointedly from asking anything which could lead to a disclosure of the diagnosis. This plea *not* to be told should be respected, although opportunities to ask questions should continue to be offered. Sometimes it is a close relative who requests that the truth be withheld – 'She's always been terrified of cancer, doctor, she'd simply give up if she knew'. Such requests are usually misguided, and most patients can come to

# R
ROSEMONT

password

g vm 2g x vA

---

l x w 6p 57v

mental health Kirby page
365, 366, NMC 6.2
Rai 7b

terms with the reality much better once it has been brought out into the open. Furthermore, a web of deceit puts family relationships under a great strain.

# Who should tell?

Ideally, this person should be a trusted and familiar doctor or nurse in the presence of a family member. However, all too often it turns out to be a stranger in the outpatient clinic or in a hospital ward.

# Breaking bad news

Although they are not very strongly evidence based, there are a few guidelines for performing this unwelcome task in a kind and courteous way.

1   Do not strive for too much detachment – patients and their relatives seem to appreciate it if the doctor or nurse is affected emotionally.
2   Try not to kill all hope, or to give a precise forecast of the duration of the illness. Offer a second opinion if one is wanted.
3   Sit down to indicate that you have time for discussion. Do not be afraid of eye contact, physical contact or silence. Describe your findings, the possible actions and the reasons for the prognosis.
4   Undertake to continue support and relieve symptoms.

# Consequent 'end-of-life decisions'

The patient may have a condition which puts a severe limit on potential *quantity* of life, such as a disseminated malignancy, a gangrenous leg or severe cardiac failure. They may have a condition which limits the potential for *quality* of life, such as end-stage dementia or an unrecovered hemiplegia. In either situation it would be reasonable to switch the emphasis of medical treatment from 'active' treatment to the relief of distressing symptoms and the preservation of dignity.

## The patient in the community

Should a medical emergency arise, the GP will need to think long and hard before sending the patient into hospital. If they decide to do so, then they will need to make it clear to the receiving doctor that the reason is to access nursing support, rather than with a view to heroic intervention. This kind of rational approach is not facilitated by the current trend towards provision of out-of-hours GP cover by on-call co-operatives.

The other problem that may be faced by GPs is exemplified by influenza immunisation. The Chief Medical Officer (and most textbooks) recommend it, for example, for patients with chronic cardiac or pulmonary disease. However, in a patient with disease that is so far advanced, an attack of influenza, preferably progressing to severe pneumonia, may be considered a merciful release.

### The hospital patient

In hospital, the usual course is to record a resuscitation status in the notes. This is sensible, because in the event of a cardiac arrest there is no time to mull over the pros and cons of cardiopulmonary resuscitation. The decision is taken by the most senior doctor available, after discussion with the rest of the team and perhaps the family. If there is any doubt, the patient is given the benefit of it. If the patient is of advanced age, it is common practice to discuss the decision with the patient, as someone aged 80 years or more might accept a very high-quality death now rather than taking his or her chances with whatever fate has in store some months or a year or two down the line.

In some ways, the emphasis that is placed on recording the patient's resuscitation status is unfortunate, as it can have the effect of pre-empting discussion of all kinds of other decisions. For example, it is not a proxy for deciding to change to palliative rather than curative treatment. A 'do not attempt resuscitation' (DNAR) decision made solely on the basis of the prognosis, for instance, should not mean depriving the patient of intravenous fluids or antibiotics.

# Living wills

Some elderly people wish to declare in advance that, in the event of serious illness and incompetence to participate in decision making due to unconsciousness or confusion, they would not wish for heroic life-supporting measures. These 'advance directives' can be drawn up on standard forms in discussion with the GP, and are regarded by the courts as imposing a strong obligation on healthcare professionals to observe their instructions. They present obvious practical difficulties. As a simple example, who will be aware of your living will if you are rushed to hospital at night as an emergency? More fundamentally, it is impossible to envisage in advance every possible medical scenario that might arise. For these reasons, some people appoint a 'health attorney' to interpret their wishes as a proxy under these circumstances. The British Medical Association has drawn up a code of practice that gives useful guidelines for preparing and implementing living wills (also *see* Chapter 8).

## Normal role of close relatives

It is obviously right for doctors to make themselves available to patients' families, and many complaints may arise from poor communication between health service staff and patients' relatives. In the case of infants, the parents have a decision-making capacity, within reasonable limits. In the case of adults, the immediate family does not, but the sensible doctor will listen attentively to their views. However, the ultimate responsibility for the decision is the doctor's. The motives of the relatives are in any case sometimes rather mixed. Those who demand that all possible life-saving measures should be taken may be riddled with guilt after years of neglecting their ailing relative. Those who suggest that it would be kinder to withdraw further aggressive treatment may be desperate to get their hands on the inheritance!

The Law Commission in the UK has proposed four tiers of decision making on behalf of incompetent adults (although legislation is still awaited):

1   the advance directive, if available
2   an attorney appointed by the patient, or a guardian appointed by a court of law
3   in the absence of any of the above, the doctor
4   where there is disagreement, the matter is to be referred to the court.

## Euthanasia

### Definitions

- *Voluntary euthanasia*: the deliberate and intentional hastening of death at the request of the patient, who is seriously ill.
- *Involuntary euthanasia*: the ending of a person's life without seeking his or her opinion.
- *Non-voluntary euthanasia*: the ending of a person's life, for his or her own benefit, when that person cannot express or cannot possess views about whether he or she lives or dies.
- *Physician-assisted suicide*: the patient takes a lethal cocktail by him- or herself which has been prescribed or provided by the physician.

### Passive and active euthanasia

The main decision confronting the doctor of a patient near the end of life is whether the aim should be palliation of symptoms or cure of the underlying cause. Most doctors subscribe to the traditional doctrine that good palliative care may involve gradually increasing the dosage of sedatives and analgesics with the aim of relieving suffering and distress, although this may have the unintended consequence of hastening the patient's death through depression of respiration, cough and movement (the so-called double effect). This is, of course, in keeping with the ruling of the House of Lords Select Committee in 1993, which concluded that it is proper to give doses of analgesic drugs and/or sedatives adequate to produce relief, even if that action has the secondary consequence of shortening life. In such cases it is the doctor's intent which is crucial. It is important to understand that increasing dosages of painkilling drugs, such as morphine, do not necessarily hasten death. Sometimes it is found that controlling the pain reduces the need for sedation and enhances the duration and quality of life.

If a patient has a gastric or colonic carcinoma that is threatening to cause obstruction, and has ascites and liver metastases, a surgeon might perform a palliative bypass procedure, but no one would expect him to carry out a radical resection, on the grounds that it would be futile. In this situation, no one would use the term 'passive euthanasia', although they might do so if the patient was not prescribed antibiotics for a postoperative chest infection that proved to be fatal. If a patient with Down's syndrome and progressive cognitive failure was denied antibiotics for pneumonia, quite a large number of people would use that expression. Passive euthanasia implies withholding or withdrawing active curative or life-prolonging treatment and allowing nature to take its course with the intention that the patient will die. It is regarded by some philosophers as morally indistinguishable from active euthanasia, but the primary intention of the doctor is critical. If it is palliation, that intention is the relief of distress, and the method used is based on a judgement of the value or futility of available treatment modalities, in the context of the patient's condition. An accurate assessment of their mental and physical condition is therefore necessary, but there is no attempt to judge the worth or futility of the patient's life. Protagonists of physician-assisted suicide talk of 'stopping treatment because a patient is dying' and 'stopping treatment because the doctor wants the patient to die', as if they were the same thing. This is not true.

The practice of active euthanasia, on the other hand, implies an intention to hasten the death of the patient on the basis of a judgement concerning the actual or potential value of his or her life, and the presumed benefit of hastening death. In the absence of a clear moral distinction between active and passive euthanasia, it is not surprising that a growing minority of UK doctors would welcome the right to help patients to end their lives in certain circumstances, either by administering a lethal injection themselves, or by handing the patient a lethal cocktail of drugs (physician-assisted suicide). Such activities are strictly against the law in the UK,* and the main argument against them is that of the

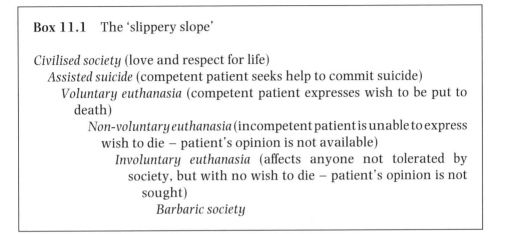

Box 11.1   The 'slippery slope'

*Civilised society* (love and respect for life)
   *Assisted suicide* (competent patient seeks help to commit suicide)
      *Voluntary euthanasia* (competent patient expresses wish to be put to
      death)
         *Non-voluntary euthanasia* (incompetent patient is unable to express
         wish to die – patient's opinion is not available)
            *Involuntary euthanasia* (affects anyone not tolerated by
            society, but with no wish to die – patient's opinion is not
            sought)
               *Barbaric society*

'slippery slope' – that is, the gradual moral decline of an entire society through actions which become increasingly corrupt due to a pervasive lack of moral insight (*see* Box 11.1). The Human Rights Act 1998 has been used on both

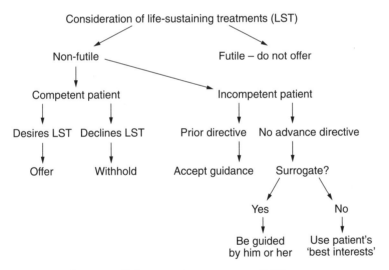

**Figure 11.1**   Consideration of life-sustaining treatments (LST).

---

* The Patient (Assisted Dying) Bill which is being debated in the House of Lords will (1) require patients to consult a doctor, a consultant physician, a psychiatrist and two witnesses, including a solicitor, (2) place a responsibility on the clinician to inform the patient of the 'alternatives, including palliative care, care in the hospice and the control of pain' and (3) stipulate a period of reflection from 7–30 days before suicide. Although the bill has passed through the second reading stage, it is unlikely to become law.

sides of the debate surrounding euthanasia. It declares a right to life, but also states that people should not be subjected to inhuman or degrading treatment, and that they should be free from torture. The courts have not interpreted this as permitting the right of competent individuals to die by active euthanasia. This was demonstrated in the case of Mrs Pretty, who had a debilitating and terminal illness. She wanted her husband to be exempt from prosecution in the event that he assisted her in ending her life. The UK courts rejected this, and the decision was upheld in Europe.

The key question that doctors are expected to ask themselves in each case is therefore 'Is the treatment worthwhile or futile?' and *not* 'Is the patient's life worthwhile or futile?'. Many would feel that some consideration of the latter question falls within the remit of a physician who is trying to act in the best interests of the patient, without justifying forms of 'treatment' or 'non-treatment' for which the primary intention is to hasten death or terminate life (*see* Figure 11.1).

# Religion

Although our society has become increasingly secular, for many people a good death will involve respect for their religious beliefs. Religion can offer some understanding of mortality. The ceremonies and rituals that surround dying can be a comfort both to patients and to their families. An understanding of religious beliefs is useful for comprehending attitudes to death, and an appreciation of these different customs is important for those involved in the care of dying patients.

Most religions promote the protection and care of those who are dying, and therefore forbid euthanasia. The monotheistic faiths, such as Christianity, Judaism and Islam, teach that life is sacred as it is given by God, and therefore ending a life is prohibited. While they teach that all life has a value, they also acknowledge that life need not be preserved at all costs. There is a recognition of the compassionate necessity to alleviate suffering and preserve dignity. As always, there is a spectrum of beliefs within these faiths. For example, the Orthodox Jewish tradition attaches much more importance to prolonging life than other faiths. In Buddhism and Hinduism there is a little more ambiguity because of the belief in reincarnation. Hastening the end of life would interfere with this process and go against the principle of *ahimsa* (doing no harm). However, there is a distinction between selfish reasons for ending life and spiritual or compassionate ones, such as the relieving of distress for relatives. These are great simplifications, but in general there is a consensus of opinion against euthanasia.

A number of case histories are given below, which illustrate some of the situations that may arise as death approaches. The patients are all elderly, representing the age group in which the large majority of deaths occur in the developed world. The real message behind these cases is that 'end-of-life' decisions are often difficult, and there may be no clear-cut right or wrong answers, but the patient's autonomy is paramount and must be respected except in cases where he or she is totally incompetent.

---

**Case 1**

Mr A, aged 82 years, was admitted with right lower lobe pneumonia. Two years previously he had a stroke and was profoundly dysarthric and unable to swallow solids or fluids without aspirating or choking. His wife had died two weeks ago, but he had an elderly dog of which he was inordinately fond. His presumed aspiration pneumonia responded well to antibiotics, but he pulled out a nasogastric tube and refused a percutaneous endoscopic gastrostomy (PEG). He wrote several pathetic notes to the medical staff begging to be allowed home. It was felt that he was not truly depressed, but that death by dehydration and starvation alone in his cold and cheerless home would be a very sad fate. After discussion with his GP, his request was acceded to, and he was doing well several months later.

**Comments**
1   The customer is always right.
2   Patients, especially the elderly, thrive far better in their own homes.

---

**Case 2**

Mrs B, aged 80 years, was admitted via the Accident and Emergency department from her residential care home where she had sustained a number of falls. Two years previously she had been diagnosed as having severe dementia, and she was now agitated and aggressive, incontinent, and variably mobile with a frame and some assistance. On his ward round, the geriatrician recorded a DNAR order in her notes. The care staff from her home reviewed her, but felt unable to have her back, so attempts were made to find a nursing-home placement. One morning Mrs B choked and aspirated, and the house officer initiated intravenous antibiotics, despite which she died. Her son subsequently complained on the grounds that:

● the DNAR decision was unjustified
● it should have been discussed with him
● it may have been made simply because we needed the bed(!).

**Comment**

A DNAR decision does not necessarily involve other non-treatment decisions unless specified.

---

**Case 3**

Mrs C, aged 78 years, who was residing in a nursing home due to multiple strokes, was sent into hospital by a visiting GP because she had ceased to eat or drink. She was profoundly dehydrated, severely dysphagic, had an indwelling catheter, and the electrolytes showed a sodium level of 183 mmol/l and a urea level of 48.9 mmol/l. She received intravenous rehydration, as the on-call team felt that this was the GP's intention and the consultant doing the 'post-take ward round' decided to send her back to the familiar surroundings of the nursing home. However, during an acrimonious interview her six sons and daughters insisted that their mother was mentally intact, valued her life, and would wish for PEG feeding, a request to which the consultant reluctantly acceded.

**Comment**

1   You are treating the patient, not the family – unless there are too many of them and they are too big and well informed!
2   Nutritional support in dysphagic stroke survivors is the most sensitive issue in the management of stroke patients. Our current strategy is to offer a nasogastric tube at 24 to 48 hours and a PEG at two weeks or so if dysphagia persists (in order to maintain nutrition rather than to protect the airway, which neither achieves), except in cases where the prognostic indicators are so bad that prolongation of life is contrary to the patient's best interest. It should be remembered that:

- loss of appetite is part of dying, so hunger is seldom a problem
- thirst is also seldom a source of suffering in clouded stroke patients
- in one study, 90% of nursing home residents with a feeding tube required restraints to stop the patients removing them
- the House of Lords recently ruled in the Tony Bland case that artificial nutrition was a treatment rather than nursing care
- similarly, the US Supreme Court ruled in the Cruzan case that artificial nutrition was a medical treatment.

Case 4

Mr D, aged 78 years, was sent into hospital with rapidly increasing breathlessness, and was found to be cachetic and to have a large pleural effusion with a 'white-out' on the X-ray. The fluid was bloodstained, but no malignant cells were found, so the respiratory physician was contacted. He suggested further aspiration for cytology and, if the result was still negative, a pleural biopsy after stopping the warfarin that Mr D was still taking for previous pulmonary emboli. This procedure was performed a week later, by which time Mr D had become progressively weaker, and he died shortly thereafter.

**Comment**
The physician's advocacy role requires him to secure the benefits of modern technology for his elderly patients – but also to have the moral courage to know when to make a clinical diagnosis and to protect the patient from over-zealous intervention.

# Summary of end-of-life decisions

1  Will further investigation clarify the overall management?
2  Information to be shared with the patient and/or their family.
3  CPR decision.
4  Is the aim of treatment curative of underlying pathology or palliation (i.e. treatment of symptoms)?
5  Against current UK law, but under intense scrutiny: deliberate termination of the patient's life if requested.

# Reference

1  Jeffery P and Millard PH (1997) An ethical framework for clinical decision-making at the end of life. *J R Soc Med.* **90**: 504–6.

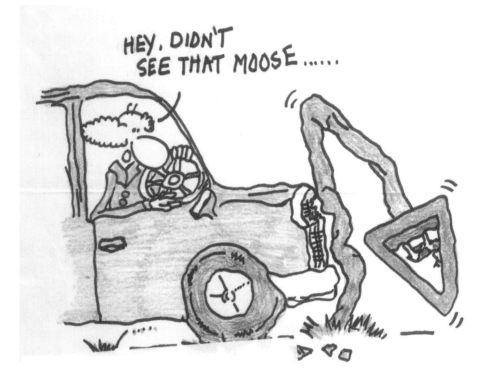

# CHAPTER 12

# Ethical issues in dementia

## Gurcharan S Rai and Iva Blackman

## Introduction

Dementia is a disease that shows increasing incidence with age. While the prevalence is about 5% in the elderly over 65 years of age, it reaches nearly 20% in those over 80 years. In clinical practice it is important to differentiate not only between acute confusional states and dementia, but also between the various types of dementia as new treatments for Alzheimer's disease become available.

Ethical issues arising in the management of dementia vary with progression of the disease. In the early stages, issues may range from questions of consent, to informing the patient that he or she has a dementing illness, to decision-making capacity. In the later stages the issues revolve around appropriate levels of care, decisions about resuscitation and end-of-life issues, financial/legal arrangements and restraining. Although there is no cure for dementia, new therapies are being developed to improve function and/or slow down the progression of disease. The recent introduction of anticholinesterase inhibitors such as donepezil, rivastigmine and gallantamine has raised the ethical issue of rationing/postcode prescribing.

Over time, alteration in a patient's cognitive state may lead to a change in the doctor–patient relationship. It is not uncommon to note that a physician, after having assessed the patient, talks to the carer as if the patient was not in the room, thus ignoring the patient's feelings. It is important for us as professionals to recognise that loss of cognitive function does not mean total loss of emotions and human values. At the very least, the physician should ensure that the patient is seen on his or her own before any discussion takes place between the doctor and the carer, and any discussion that takes place should involve the patient.

## Ethical issues in the early stages of dementia

In the early stages, patients with dementia have the capacity to undertake decisions with regard to their treatment (i.e. choose to accept or refuse), and therefore should not be treated any differently from other patients and should be allowed to exercise that choice. Denying choice compromises independence and dignity. In the USA, some recommend that this is the opportune time for the patient with dementia to be encouraged to draw up an advance directive which, as stated by the High Court in patient C, is a binding document if prepared by a mentally competent person. This process will of course only succeed if:

1   there is frank and open discussion between the patient, his or her family and the physician, and
2   the patient is given a full explanation of advance directives and about the medical care that he or she is likely to receive at various stages of the illness.

# Informing the patient about the diagnosis

It is argued by some that because dementia is a progressive disease with no available curative treatment, some patients will be unable to accept the diagnosis, and as a result may suffer psychological distress with a subsequent reduction in hope and motivation. Although it is true that, in practice, some patients find it difficult to accept a diagnosis with a poor prognosis (e.g. they switch off during discussion), it should be possible to discuss the diagnosis sympathetically, providing support to the patient over two or more sessions. Basic principles require that we as physicians should be honest and tell the patient the truth so that they can exercise their moral and ethical right to decide, while they are still competent, whether they wish to accept or reject treatment or investigations should they become incompetent. This may also lead to patients accepting the involvement of support groups or help from psychologists and community psychiatric nurses. This in turn helps through discussion to overcome psychological reactions of fear, depression and anger. In addition, patients may also decide to seek guidance about advance directives.

In some cases, family members may insist that a patient should not be informed of the diagnosis. Under these circumstances it is important to clarify that a competent individual has the moral and legal right to know the diagnosis and make decisions about their future care, which also includes treatment.

# Informing family/carers about the diagnosis

Family members may not only ask for the diagnosis to be kept from the patient, but may also ask for the diagnosis to be given to them before it is given to the patient. In the latter situation it is important to inform the family that doctors cannot, either in law or ethically, give information to a third party without the consent and agreement of a competent adult (i.e. the patient). In fact, a competent patient can ask a doctor not to talk to a particular family member, and if this happens, doctors must act in accordance with the patient's wishes. Of course in the late stages of dementia when the patient is unlikely to have the capacity to give consent, the doctor should talk to the family. Sharing information with the family and carer involved in providing support and care to the patient will not only help the doctor to obtain insight into the patient's past wishes, but will also ensure that appropriate care is organised in the best interests of the patient.

# Issues surrounding genetics

Recent developments in genetics have identified mutations that predispose to Alzheimer's disease on chromosomes 21,14, 19 and 1. The gene located on chromosome 21, an autosomal-dominant gene, was the first to be discovered in groups of families in whom the onset of dementia started at below the age of 65 years. This gene results in the production of a precursor protein B-amyloid around plaques. The genetic abnormality on chromosome 19, the second to be discovered, represents a risk factor for individuals over the age of 60 years. The allele associated with increased risk is e4. The third abnormal gene located on chromosome 14 (an autosomal-dominant gene) is responsible for 70–80% of familial cases. The fourth gene locus on chromosome 1 relates to an early onset of familial dementia. Although chromosome 1 is a dominant gene, at least two examples of probable incomplete penetrance have been identified. The three Alzheimer's disease genes (chromosomes 21, 14 and 1) account for fewer than 5% of all cases. Therefore in the majority of patients with Alzheimer's dementia it is a polygenic multifactorial disorder in which some gene effects may be found, but environmental and other modulatory factors may be of central importance.

Although some physicians and relatives may suggest or demand screening for families, particularly for those with familial Alzheimer's disease, the majority reject it on the grounds that there is no preventative or protective treatment currently available, and that it has the additional disadvantage of causing psychological trauma for the individual and their family. The Nuffield Council on Bioethics has advised against the introduction of genetic testing in disorders/diseases with multiple causes, and thus this applies to most if not all older patients with Alzheimer's disease. However, if a doctor agrees to the demand for genetic testing from a member of the family of a patient with familial Alzheimer's disease, counselling before and after testing is regarded as essential.

# Ethical issues surrounding new treatment

At the present time there are four drugs available for use in patients with Alzheimer's disease, namely donepezil (a piperidine-based reversible inhibitor of acetylcholinesterase), rivastigmine (a centrally selective inhibitor of acetylcholinesterase), gallantamine (a competitive acetylcholinesterase inhibitor) and memantine (a voltage-dependent, moderate-affinity non-competitive NMDA-receptor antagonist). Donepezil, rivastigmine and gallantamine are recommended for patients with mild to moderate dementia, and memantine is recommended for patients with the later stages of the disease. None of these drugs is curative, and not all patients with Alzheimer's disease show a response to them.

The introduction of these drugs has not met with universal enthusiasm from health authorities, and there is evidence that some of them are refusing to fund this treatment, quoting cost as one of the factors that has influenced their decision. Cost, of course, also raises the issue about the ethics of pharmaceutical companies who charge a high price for a drug in order to make a profit for the shareholders.

Although it is reasonable not to offer treatment that is deemed futile, it is ethically (and may now be legally) wrong to deny treatment on the grounds of cost alone, if that treatment has been shown to be of benefit. In a recent ruling on a case involving a patient with multiple sclerosis who was denied interferon treatment, the judge stated that the policy adopted by the health authority was 'the very antithesis' of NHS guidelines, and that the drug should be given to 'those who need it most'.

The other ethical issue in relation to prescribing of anti-dementia drugs is that of consent. In UK law, an adult is presumed to have the capacity to make decisions and to act upon those decisions. Therefore it follows that before an anti-dementia drug can be prescribed, a doctor must obtain the patient's consent. However, significant numbers of patients with dementia are incapable of giving consent, and if the ethical guidelines on consent to treatment are strictly adhered to, many of these patients would be wrongly deprived of treatment from which they could benefit. Therefore it is accepted practice that if patients cannot give consent to medical treatment, the doctor should act in the patient's best interest after full consideration of the benefits and unwanted effects of the treatment, and after full consultation with the family/carers who know the patient best.

# Issues surrounding patients' liberty to drive

Dementia can lead not only to changes in memory but also to impairment of judgement, visuospatial difficulties and inattentiveness. All of these changes can affect driving, and there is evidence that a diagnosis of dementia is associated with an increased risk of accidents. Patients with Alzheimer's dementia are five times more likely to have a car accident than their age-matched health controls. This raises the following questions.

1 What advice should doctors give to patients with dementia?
2 What should happen if patients continue to drive against their doctor's wishes?
3 What is the law regarding fitness to drive?

# What advice should doctors give to patients with dementia?

The answer to this question should be based on a full assessment of the patient, since not all patients with a diagnosis of dementia become unfit to drive at the time when the diagnosis is made. In the early stages there may not be any gross difficulties with judgement, visual perception, visuospatial discrimination or attention. Under these circumstances, patients can be advised that they may continue to drive until difficulties start to arise. However, if the patient admits to difficulties, a carer reports difficulties or the patient has a moderate degree of dementia, then that patient should be advised not to drive until a full assessment has been made. This may involve psychometric assessment by a psychologist and assessment by driver licensing authorities (such as the DVLA in the UK) to determine their medical fitness to hold a licence. The initial assessment by the DVLA consists of a medical enquiry about the patient addressed to his or her GP regarding episodes of confusion or memory problems. In addition, they may ask for reports from consultant psychiatrists or an independent medical assessment and psychometric report. If doubt remains after this assessment, a full assessment may take place at a recognised Disabled Driver Assessment Unit, where physical and psychometric assessments are undertaken. If doubt about the person's ability to drive still persists, they may be asked to take a full driving test.

Finally, it is important to note that simple cognitive tests such as the Mini-Mental State Examination are very poor predictors of driving ability.

# What should happen if patients continue to drive against their doctor's wishes?

It is important for us, as doctors, first to remember that we have a legal duty to respect the confidence of a patient, and secondly not only to consider the right of a person with dementia to maintain their personal freedom, but also to consider the right of everyone to be safe. Although reporting of suspected medical unfitness to drive raises an important ethical dilemma about confidentiality, most physicians now accept that the principle of confidentiality is partly or wholly balanced by a 'common good' principle for the protection of third parties. In the UK, the doctor only informs the DVLA in Swansea directly on failure to persuade the person to do this him- or herself, and when the doctor has grounds to suspect that the patient is at risk.

# What is the law regarding fitness to drive?

In the UK, the 1988 Road Traffic Act and the more recent Motor Vehicles (Driver Licences) Regulations 1996 define severe mental disorders as a relevant disability for licensing, and this includes dementia. The person is obliged by law to inform the DVLA about his/her condition. If a patient refuses to do this despite advice from their doctor and family, the doctor can inform the DVLA directly after first informing the patient of this decision.

# Ethical problems associated with the late stages of dementia

As the disease progresses, patients become increasingly less able to make decisions. However, this does not imply incompetence. Although they may not understand the benefits and risks of medical intervention, they may still be able to understand their finances or home circumstances. Therefore it is essential that competence is assessed in the area in question.

# Treatment of acute illness, including decisions about resuscitation

As the disease progresses, patients become mentally incompetent and therefore unable to make decisions about treatment. Under these circumstances, unless the patient has left an advance directive or a living will, doctors should make decisions on behalf of the patient, after talking to his or her friends and carers with the aim of finding out what decision the patient would have made while competent. If this is not possible, as in the majority of cases, doctors should make a decision in the 'best interest' of the patient.

It is recommended that when considering what is in the best interest of the patient, regard should be paid to the following:

1   the prognosis
2   the ascertainable past and present wishes and feelings of the person con-
    cerned, and the factors that person would consider if he or she were able to
    do so
3   the views of other people whom it is appropriate and practicable to consult
    about the patient's wishes and feelings and what would be in his or her best
    interest
4   whether the purpose for which any action or decision is required can be effec-
    tively achieved in a manner that is less restrictive of the person's freedom.

This decision-making process may involve looking at the benefits as well as the
risks/burdens/side-effects of treatment, the quality of life of the patient prior to
their becoming ill, and the likely quality of life on recovery. Since quality of life
is difficult to assess, it would be acceptable to make a judgement based on the
severity of the disease. Some argue that 'once a person is unable to recognise
loved ones then that person has reached a stage where the meaning of human
life has deteriorated and death is inevitable'. It therefore becomes acceptable
not to offer life-sustaining treatment. Symptomatic relief such as antipyretics
for fever, mouth care, bowel care to prevent constipation, bladder care to prevent retention of urine, and skin care to prevent pressure sores are deemed
reasonable to administer. This concept is consistent with the accepted principle
that doctors have a duty to ensure that death is achieved without pain and
with dignity. In this situation, resuscitation should not be performed.

# Percutaneous endoscopic gastrostomy (PEG) feeding

---

**Case 1**

An 85-year-old woman who has severe Alzheimer's disease is admitted to
hospital from a nursing home with right lower lobe pneumonia. Assessment by a speech and language therapist revealed poor swallowing on
admission to hospital. Nurses start her on nasogastric feeding. During the
next seven days the patient pulls out the nasogastric tube on six occasions.

  After the seven days, when her clinical features of pneumonia have
improved, the question of PEG is raised. The speech and language therapist
feels that the patient is unlikely to pull out her PEG as it does not normally
cause discomfort.

---

Swallowing problems are not uncommon in patients with dementia with the progression of disease, and particularly at times of acute illness. In some the ability to swallow returns, while in others the swallowing difficulties remain, making oral intake unsafe. At this stage PEG may be considered and discussed as a long-term option between the members of the multi-disciplinary team and the family. Often the question of whether it is appropriate to place a PEG tube in a severely demented patient will be asked.

This dilemma is not uncommonly encountered by doctors who are caring for older people. In decision making, the doctor should consider the following:

1  the benefits and risks associated with PEG in this group of patients. Data from one large study suggest that tube feeding patients with advanced dementia does not prevent aspiration pneumonia, prolong survival, reduce the risk of pressure sores or improve function and comfort. In addition, PEG is associated with local irritation, which can lead to potentially fatal complications. The majority of the frail elderly do not survive one year after the procedure

2  the benefits and risks associated with PEG in the patient concerned. Comorbidity in an individual increases the risk of complications, particularly mortality

3  whether the patient has left instructions in the form of a living will, or if no living will has been made, discuss the matter with their close family members or carers to discover the patient's previously expressed values, and try to judge how the patient would have responded to the offer of a PEG had he or she been fully competent. Here it is important to remember that in England, Wales and Northern Ireland the family cannot make a proxy decision, whereas in Scotland a person who has been given the power of attorney has the right to make decisions on behalf of a patient who has become mentally incompetent

4  discussion with the staff involved in caring for the patient of the benefits and risks of PEG feeding

5  assessment of the patient's present behaviour. Are they trying to indicate that they do not wish to be fed by pulling out nasogastric tubes repeatedly or by declining to take food orally when it is offered?

After consideration and full discussion with the family/carers and other members of staff involved in providing care for the patient, a decision in the best interests of the patient should be made, remembering that artificial feeding is regarded as medical treatment and as such does not need to be offered to a patient who is in the terminal/final stages of dementia, or who is unlikely to benefit. Finally, it should be noted that in some patients with dementia dysphagia may not be part and parcel of the expected decline in dementia, and may in fact be the result of another illness. Under these circumstances it would be appropriate to offer PEG feeding.

# Use of physical and chemical restraints

Personality and behavioural changes are common with progression of the disease process. Aberrant behaviour with or without wandering, particularly in the presence of an acute illness, may become a major problem for the patient's carer/family as well as for professionals who are providing help and care for those affected by the disease. Although it would be wrong to restrain someone physically (and in the UK it is against the law) or chemically just for the benefit of carers or hospital staff, it should be considered where it is in the best interest of the patient. One should take the caregiver's stress into consideration in the decision-making process. The proposed ethical guidelines devised by the Ethics and Humanities Subcommittee of the American Academy of Neurology include the following.

1   Restraints should be ordered when they contribute to the safety of the patient or others and are not simply a convenience for the staff.
2   Restraints should not be ordered as a substitute for careful evaluation and surveillance of the patient, as appropriate for good medical practice.
3   The perceived need for restraints should trigger medical assessment and investigation of the precise reason for them, intended to correct the underlying medical or psychological problem.
4   If a proxy decision maker is known, restraints should be ordered after full discussion of the risks and benefits. However, in an acute situation doctors should act in the best interest of the patient.
5   When they are indicated, pharmacological agents should be used at the lowest dose possible.
6   All restraints should be reassessed frequently so that they may be in effect for the shortest duration necessary to achieve their goals.

# Use of monitoring equipment

Assistive technology continues to develop not only in order to enable independence for the elderly but also for the purpose of monitoring the well-being of an individual. Video and electronic tags are now widely available and are being employed by some institutions and private homes for monitoring elderly patients with dementia, who have a tendency to wander and a predisposition to fall. There is no doubt that the use of such equipment raises issues such as freedom/liberty, and it is therefore important that any decision to use them takes into account such important issues and places the individual older person at the centre of the decision-making process. The final decision should be based on the principle of 'best interest' of the older person, and not on the interest of the staff/carer or the home itself.

# Law and financial handling capacity of patients with dementia

As dementia progresses, patients become increasingly less able to handle their financial affairs. In the early stages an individual can ask another person to help collect a pension or pay bills on the odd occasion. However, for permanent arrangements the patient with dementia who has the capacity to understand and make decisions should be advised to make an *enduring power of attorney*.

Enduring power of attorney was introduced in England and Wales in 1985. It covers financial matters but not decisions on medical treatment or non-financial personal arrangements. It may give 'general' authority to carry out all transactions on behalf of the individual, or specific authority. This gives the person authority to sign cheques or withdraw money from the bank. This is achieved by completing the form of enduring power of attorney which is available from stationers that supply legal forms.

In the late stages of dementia, when the patient loses the mental capacity to manage his or her affairs, the enduring power of attorney loses its validity and the attorney must apply to register the enduring power of attorney with the Court of Protection before he or she can act or continue to act under it. This means that the grantor and certain stipulated close relatives must then be informed, and they are given the right to object. The Court of Protection can terminate the enduring power of attorney if the appointed attorney is found to be dishonest or becomes mentally incapable.

When there is no enduring power of attorney, the Court of Protection should be considered if the patient is not capable of managing his or her affairs because of mental incapacity, or if there is dispute among the family members as to who should handle the patient's financial affairs. The Court of Protection relates to financial matters, and can be asked to write a will for the incapacitated person if no will exists, or to supersede an existing will if it is no longer appropriate.

# What about those who neglect themselves at home because of dementia but refuse to accept help?

In the late stages of dementia, personal neglect is not only common but often denied by the patient. Commonly this information becomes available when a person is admitted to hospital with an acute illness. A dilemma arises, with conflict between autonomy and beneficence, when the patient recovers from the physical illness and insists on going home. The individual's wishes (patient's autonomy) must be respected. Actions must be taken to reduce or minimise neglect as far as possible through discussion with the patient, their family/ carers and all of the agencies involved in providing community services. If this is not possible, and the patient refuses to accept help or to leave home to go into a safer environment (and from assessment it is clear that the patient is unable to understand the risks of going home), then in the UK 'guardianship' under the Mental Health Act 1983 can be exercised in order to ensure the welfare of the patient and the protection of others. This will allow the patient to be moved to a safer environment. To enforce this section, the signatures of two registered practitioners (one of whom should be a specialist) are required.

The other sections of the Mental Health Act can also be used to detain patients with dementia. For example, under Section 4 a person can be admitted as an emergency if the relatives and social workers cannot cope with the patient's behaviour. The period of detention under the section is a maximum of 72 hours, but this can be changed to 28 days by seeking a specialist opinion.

Section 47 of the National Assistance Act 1948 can also be used to admit a person to hospital who is unable to care for himself at home, not receiving care at home, suffering from a grave chronic disease or living in unsanitary conditions. This act does not allow treatment to be given against the patient's wishes. The other drawback, of course, is the fact that unlike the Mental Health Act 1983 it does not provide safeguards for the person with respect to review procedures.

# Abuse of the elderly with dementia

Mental impairment makes the elderly vulnerable to abuse, which may take the form of physical, mental and financial abuse as well as deprivation of nutrition, help in activities of daily living and prescribed drugs. Recognition of abuse can be difficult because physical changes may mimic the changes of ageing and the elderly person may be unwilling or unable to admit to abuse.

Although it may be possible if a person is in an institution to take action through statutory bodies that visit institutions, it is difficult to take action against a relative/carer who is suspected of abuse if the elderly person is unwilling or unable to co-operate. This raises the important ethical issue of whether action should be taken against the wishes of an elderly person in order to protect them. Unfortunately, there is no law that allows professionals to make the elderly Wards of Court, as is the case with children. Therefore we have no option but to work closely with all of the professionals involved in providing care for the older person. This also includes relatives, who unfortunately may themselves be the abusers of the elderly patient. It is hoped that vigilant and consistent contact will reduce the likelihood of abuse. To help with this process, local health authorities and social services have drawn up guidelines for staff to follow.

---

**Key points**

- In the early stages, patients with dementia have the full capacity to undertake decision making with regard to their treatment, and therefore should not be treated differently from other patients.
- Basic principles require the physician to tell the patient that he or she has dementia.
- Since there are no available preventative or therapeutic agents that can cure dementia, it is not necessary to carry out genetic testing to establish whether a family member has the gene or not.
- Any new effective treatment that is developed should be offered to patients, and no one should be denied treatment solely on the grounds of cost.
- Patients with obvious impairment of judgement or visuospatial difficulties should be asked to stop driving. If they fail to take this advice, they should be reported to the Driver and Vehicle Licensing Agency, even if it means breaking the rule about patient confidentiality.
- In the late stages of disease, doctors may have to make decisions about which treatment is best for the individual. In end-stage dementia, when the patient is unable to recognise loved ones, life-sustaining treatment need not be offered but palliative care should be practised instead.
- Chemical restraints should only be used if they contribute to the safety of the patient or others, not simply for the convenience of staff.
- In the early stages of dementia, patients should be encouraged to consider enduring power of attorney, which can then be registered with the Court of Protection when the patient becomes mentally incapable.
- Patients who neglect themselves may have to be admitted to hospital under Section 47 of the National Assistance Act, or moved into a residential home using guardianship under the Mental Health Act 1983.

---

# Further reading

- American Academy of Neurology, Ethics and Humanities Subcommittee (1996) Ethical issues in the management of the demented patient. *Neurology*. **46**: 1180–3.

- Arie T (1996) Some legal aspects of mental capacity. *BMJ*. **313**: 156–8.

- Finucane TE, Christmas C and Travis K (1999) Tube feeding in patients with advanced dementia. A review of the evidence. *JAMA*. **282**: 1365–70.

- National Institute for Clinical Excellence (2001) *Guidance on the use of Donepezil, Rivastigmine and Gallantamine for the treatment of Alzheimer's disease*. Technology Appraisal Guidance No. 19 (www.nice.org.uk)

- Post SG (1994) Alzheimer's disease – ethics and progression of dementia. *Clin Geriatr Med.* **10**: 379–94.

- Post SG and Whitehouse PJ (1995) Fairhill Guidelines on ethics of the care of people with Alzheimer's disease: a clinical summary. *J Am Geriatr Soc.* **43**: 1423–9.

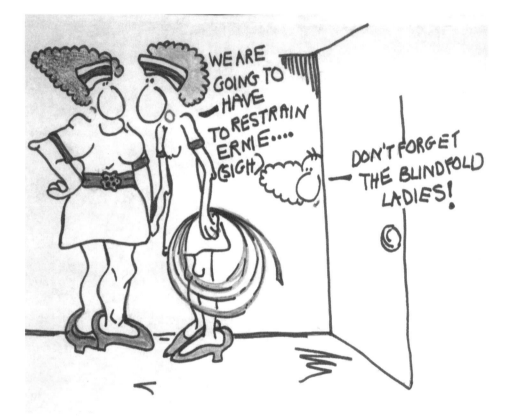

# CHAPTER 13

# The use of restraints

## Nick Coni and Gurcharan S Rai

## Introduction

Good clinical practice demands that we show respect for the autonomy of patients. Despite this, various types of restraints which limit the freedom of movement continue to be used, often without the patient's consent. The published data suggest a high prevalence rate (approximately 36%) for use of physical restraints in nursing homes, despite the absence of objective data demonstrating their effectiveness. In fact, evidence from empirical research suggests that restrained residents in a nursing-home setting may show more agitated behaviour and suffer adverse effects such as chronic constipation, incontinence, pressure sores, sensory deprivation, reduced functional capacity and dependency. Institutions justify the use of restraints on the grounds that it is their duty to protect those under their care from harm, and also their duty to respect the autonomy of other people.

The moral and ethical dilemmas associated with the use of restraints raise two important issues. First, institutions must set up standards of care on the use of restraints that balance the importance of the patient's freedom and their requirement to safeguard the patient. Secondly, each professional who advocates the use of restraints must establish the justification for their use and try to obtain consent from the proxy decision maker for a patient who is not competent to make a decision him- or herself. Having said that, it is important for all institutions to have the aim of practising restraint-free care, and with this objective some have already developed alternative methods, such as listening to preferred music, to produce positive behaviours in the institutionalised confused elderly.

In the USA, the OBRA '87 guidelines, included in the Nursing Home Reform Amendments of the Omnibus Budget Reconciliation Act of 1987, state that:

1   the resident has the right to be free from any physical restraints imposed for the purpose of discipline or convenience, and that are not required to treat the resident's medical condition

2   the nursing home is obliged to demonstrate that less restrictive methods have been tried

3   physical and occupational therapists are consulted prior to using the restraints.

In addition to the harmful effects of restraints, it is worth remembering that a restraining environment is non-rehabilitative and non-therapeutic.

In the case of chemical restraints, the OBRA '87 regulations state that:

1   residents should have a comprehensive assessment prior to the use of anti-psychotic drugs

2   residents who have not used antipsychotic drugs are not given them unless antipsychotic drug therapy is necessary to treat a specific condition

3   residents who use antipsychotic drugs receive gradual dose reductions and behavioural interventions, unless these are clinically contraindicated.

Since the introduction of the OBRA '87 guidelines, there have been studies showing a significant reduction in the number of falls with injuries with the removal of physical barriers.

# Use of restraints in institutions

Patients in hospital wards and nursing homes find themselves in a strange environment surrounded by unfamiliar faces. They readily become disorientated, especially if they are vulnerable due to cognitive impairment, impaired vision or hearing, acute physical disease, or medication or its sudden withdrawal. This may lead to a tendency to get up and wander, or to disturbed and aggressive behaviour. Discomfort due to pain, an impacted rectum or full bladder is likely to precipitate an attempt to wander, or the patient may simply be motivated by boredom or a very understandable wish to escape. Many of these patients will be unsteady on their feet, and here again poor vision, strange surroundings, physical illness and medication are very likely to make matters worse. It is therefore not surprising that falls are quite common in institutions. Falls are 'bad' for the health – they lead to fractured hips (and wrists, vertebrae, ribs and pubic rami), subdural haematomata, bruising and lacerations, and complaints against the staff and threatened or actual litigation. A natural reaction by the staff is to become overprotective and seek to prevent such incidents through the use of restraints. Restraints are also used for other reasons – for instance, to prevent patients from wandering off and getting lost or becoming exposed to danger, or to prevent them from invading other patients' space and causing them distress. Restraints come in various forms, and almost all of them are undesirable.

# Physical restraints: personal

These include the use of cot-sides at night in case the occupant falls out of bed. People generally do not fall out of bed – they fall while getting out of bed – so the provision of cot-sides ensures that the fall occurs from a greater height (by half a metre or so more than it otherwise would). This certainly applies to confused, restless but reasonably agile patients. More lethargic, frail subjects may receive some protection from the fitting of cot-sides, because they sometimes slither from the side of the bed to the floor and an obstacle may remind them to ask for help with going to the toilet. A rather less forbidding form of restraint is the 'cocoon', which is formed by zipping the sides of the duvet to the valance.

Personal restraints also include imprisoning patients in tilting chairs with trays across the front, which become very uncomfortable. The use of tilting chairs and cot-sides is now avoided by nurses in the UK, except as a last resort, although this is not the case in a number of other countries. Unfortunately, the prevention of falls in institutions for the frail and dependent without recourse to restraints often requires higher staffing levels than those currently provided, and may be impossible to achieve when trying to give adequate protection to confused patients. The ever-present threat of complaint and litigation has also had a malign influence on risk management in this context.

Rather more controversial is the use of electronic tagging, whereby a device strapped to the wrist sets off an alarm if the patient leaves the hospital ward. This is regarded by some as an infringement of the patient's civil liberties. Unfortunately, the disorientated person who strolls off the ward, turns left into intensive care and starts to disconnect the various life-support systems of a critical road traffic accident victim is interfering with another patient's civil liberties – as well as being vulnerable to electrocution.

A final mention should perhaps be made of the occasional necessity for tying patients' limbs, either to permit the administration of essential medication or to prevent self-harm. Examples might include a chlormethiazole infusion for status epilepticus, when the arm providing venous access is splinted, or the patient who tears at already damaged skin, when the hands are bandaged. The subjects are invariably acutely confused and generally clouded, and the intention is for such measures to be used only in the very short term while the underlying condition is treated and normal cerebral function is hopefully restored. In some countries it is common practice to use mittens for those who repeatedly pull out their nasogastric tubes or catheters. It is important to remember that whenever mittens are employed in this way their use is fully discussed within the multi-professional team and, more importantly, their benefit is clearly documented in the patient's records.

# Physical restraints: environmental

During the 1950s and 1960s a wave of enlightenment swept through our mental hospitals, and the doors which had been slammed shut by their Victorian governors were flung open by the pioneers of post-war psychiatry. Some doors were opened wider than others, and it is still common to find wards with doors that are unlocked, but which can only be opened by operating a higher ('baffle') catch at the same time as the one at the normal level. This manoeuvre is not readily learned by demented patients. One problem which arises here is how to advise the relatives or neighbours of a confused elderly person who lives at home but tends to wander into the road in her nightie in the middle of the night. A similar device might constitute an obstacle to escape in the event of a fire. Another infringement of liberty that is nevertheless sometimes essential for safety in the home is to disconnect the kitchen gas and electrical appliances, or even to blockade access to the kitchen.

# Chemical restraints

The use of sedatives and tranquillisers was condemned long ago as a 'pharmacological straitjacket', and should be kept to a minimum, although it must be admitted that it does occasionally seem to be justified for very noisy, disruptive patients on a general ward, largely for the sake of the other patients. It is preferable by far to identify and treat the cause of such behaviour, or failing that to secure a more appropriate type of care for such patients, but unfortunately this is not always possible. The use of these drugs is very often counter-productive for the reasons listed in Table 13.1.

The law permits a hospital doctor to prescribe an injection of a tranquilliser and to summon porters to hold down a severely agitated patient while the nurse

**Table 13.1**   Adverse effects of benzodiazepines, butyrophenones and especially phenothiazines when used for confused, wandering patients

| Effect | Result |
| --- | --- |
| Impaired psychomotor function | Increased sway, increased liability to fall |
| Sedation | Increased liability to fall |
| Postural hypotension | Increased liability to fall |
| Extrapyramidal side-effects | Increased liability to fall |
| Reduced movements | Pressure sores |
| Restlessness, confusion on withdrawal | Problem worsened |

administers it, when it is for the patient's own protection. In the case of confused elderly people, this causes a great deal of distress to one and all – except, quite often, the patient. However, the Mental Health Act 1983 specifically provides for mentally disordered patients to be given treatment for their own safety and protection without their consent.

# The Coroner and deaths following falls

A death caused by a fall is an accidental death, and as such should be reported to the Coroner. On the other hand, a tendency to fall is a part of the natural history of many age-related disorders, and many patients will have sustained numerous falls in the weeks or months before their deaths which have contributed to their poor mobility, their chair- or bed-bound state, their venous thromboses and their hypostatic pneumonias, and these do not need to be referred to the Coroner. In between are those deaths which ensue several weeks after surgery for a fractured femoral neck, and the sharp dip which this so often represents in a pre-existing inexorable functional decline. The only golden rule here is if in doubt, discuss it with the Coroner's officer, who will almost certainly give an extremely sensible ruling.

---

**Case 1**

Mr G is in his early seventies and is in hospital waiting for a place in a facility for the 'elderly mentally infirm'. He has diabetes and has developed extremely painful ulcers on both heels, which require surgical debridement. His normal restlessness is exacerbated by the pain, and he is continually getting out of bed at night and falling. As he is in a single room to avoid disruption to the other patients, he cannot be under constant surveillance, so the nurses have removed the bed and put the mattress on the floor, where he is relatively comfortable.

---

**Case 2**

At the time of his final admission to a predominantly non-acute geriatric hospital, while his wife received urgent treatment in another hospital, Mr P was 85 years of age and physically fairly robust, although demented.

Late one evening he left his ward, opened the safety gate at the top of the stairs, descended the single flight of stairs to the ground floor, and clambered over the safety gate at the bottom. He walked through a ground-floor ward, refused to allow a nurse to sit him down and bring him a cup of tea, opened the fire doors at the end of the ward, which opened on to a balcony, climbed over a safety fence and fell several feet into a flower bed. As a result he sustained a crush fracture of a lumbar vertebra. Over the next three months his pain required strong analgesia and his loss of mobility led to pressure sores, dehydration, urinary tract infection and episodes of septicaemia. Eventually it was decided to focus medical and nursing endeavours on alleviating his suffering and allowing him to die with dignity.

Mrs P and her children expressed strong dissatisfaction with the care and surveillance exercised by the staff, and with the security and suitability of the building for its present purpose, and took legal advice. However, expert opinion maintained that it was not modern practice to confine such patients within cot-sides or to administer sedatives if at all possible to prevent wandering, although the level of staffing should perhaps be examined. As there were no previous reports of accidents resulting from falls from this particular balcony, it would be difficult to establish that the hospital was negligent in the design of the safety railings surrounding it.

Most importantly, although with the wisdom of hindsight Mr P's disturbed behaviour had in fact been a danger to himself, the nurses could not be regarded as failing in their duty of care for not recognising this at the time and using physical force to restrain him, as such force is now avoided, if at all possible, because it usually causes distress and increased agitation and aggression.

**Case 3**

During an earlier admission, Mr G had become abruptly confused, agitated and aggressive, and was brandishing his stick, shaking the windows and impossible to calm. Hypoglycaemia having been excluded (with difficulty), he was forcibly injected with haloperidol 5 mg, which was repeated twice. After sleeping it off, he was docile and co-operative and remembered nothing of the incident. He was discharged home with a diagnosis of probable early dementia, which did not become incapacitating until two years later.

**Key points**

- It is important for each of us as individuals to have freedom of movement. Therefore no one should advocate returning to the use of physical restraints of the straitjacket type. In addition, the use of physical restraints in the UK is against the law.
- Although it is morally unjustifiable to restrain patients, especially when there is empirical research data to suggest that this is associated with adverse effects, there will always be a small number of patients who, because of their agitation or tendency to wander, require restriction for their own safety.
- In the hospital setting, it is essential that the hospital sets standards of care with regard to the use of restraints that balance the importance of the patient's freedom with the requirement of the hospital to safeguard the patient.
- Each individual professional who advocates the use of restraint must first establish the justification for its use and secondly, if possible, try to obtain consent from the proxy decision maker for a patient who is not competent to make a decision him- or herself.
- Where restraint is required as a best course of care, it may be justified without the patient's consent if the patient lacks sufficient autonomy to make any choice.
- Law permits a hospital doctor to prescribe an injection of a tranquilliser and to summon porters to hold down a severely agitated patient while the nurse administers it, when this is for the patient's own protection.

# Further reading

- Dodds S (1996) Exercising restraint: autonomy, welfare and elderly patients. *J Med Ethics.* **22**: 160–3.

- Elton R and Pawlson LG (1992) The impact of OBRA on medical practice within nursing facilities. *J Am Geriatr Soc.* **40**: 958–63.

- Frank C, Hodgetts G and Puxty J (1966) Safety and efficacy of physical restraints for the elderly. Review of the evidence. *Can Fam Physician.* **42**: 2402–9.

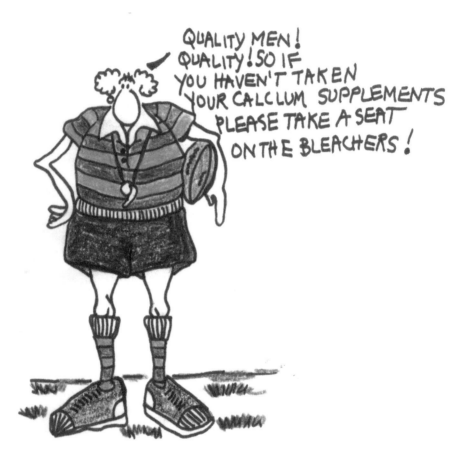

# CHAPTER 14

# Quality of life in healthcare decisions

## Ann Bowling

## Introduction: quality of life vs. length of life

Research in the USA indicates that patients have expressed a preference for survival for a shorter life of improved quality.[1,2] However, research on cancer patients in the UK has shown that most patients would accept toxic chemotherapy for minimal benefit in relation to prolongation of life.[3] The issue is further complicated by research in the USA which has shown that most patients in geriatric wards indicated that they wanted to be resuscitated if their heart stopped beating, while few of their doctors had marked them for resuscitation in the medical notes.[4] It appears that doctors often rate the quality of life of the patient as lower than the patient perceives it, and the life itself of lower value than the patient rates it. The only way to face ethical dilemmas about treatments is to *ask the patient* about their perception of their quality of life and their treatment preferences.

## Age-related treatment policies

Negative assumptions about the quality of life of elderly people, together with a general ageism in Western society, have led to age cut-off points for treatments, which are not based on the evidence of clinical effectiveness, in some health districts. This is apparent, for example, in cardiology in relation to access to rehabilitation centres, cardiological investigations and specific, clinically effective treatments (e.g. revascularisation through coronary artery bypass graft [CABG][5]). However, increasingly the literature on health-related quality of life does not justify age-related policies. For example, a five-year follow-up study of the broader quality of life of 1371 patients aged over 74 years at operation (mean age at operation 77 years) and 257 'neutral-risk' patients (mean age at operation 58 years), all of whom were undergoing CABG, reported that CABG is justified in very elderly people because the *health-related quality* of the extended survival was as good as that reported for younger patients and that for age-adjusted populations.[6] Although few clinical trials of treatments currently include patients aged over 65 or 70 years, it is important to measure the effects of treatments in older people as well as in younger subjects. This is more pertinent with the ageing of the population, and evidence of a healthier older population than in the past, together with the emphasis on positive ageing and equal rights to appropriate and clinically effective treatments among all age groups.

Although over-investigation and medical intervention to prolong life at the expense of quality of life at any age merit ethical debate, and while any mortality risk must be balanced against the potential gains in life years and in quality of life, it is important to ensure equal access to clinically effective and appropriate treatments from which older as well as younger people can benefit in the broadest sense.

# Measuring health-related quality of life

Such studies indicate the value of measuring health-related quality of life when assessing the outcome of clinical interventions. The broader measurement of *health outcome* has become a cornerstone of health services research. Purchasers of healthcare want to know what *health gain* interventions provide. This emphasis is positive, and health-related quality of life assessment is increasingly incorporated into criteria for the assessment of people's needs for effective services. Treatments and interventions need to be evaluated in terms of whether they are more likely to lead to an outcome of *a life worth living* in social, psychological and physical terms, and people themselves are the best judges of this in relation to their own lives.

Health-related quality of life is a subjective concept, and relates to the perceived effects of health status on the ability to live a fulfilling life. This encompasses functional ability in relation to ability to perform self-care tasks, domestic tasks and mobility, role functioning (e.g. ability to function in work, social roles such as parenting, etc.), the existence and quality of relationships and social interaction, psychological well-being (e.g. life satisfaction, adjustment, coping ability), autonomy and control, and mental health (e.g. anxiety, depression, cognitive state). As with the concept, the potential range of dimensions of health-related quality of life which could be measured in studies of health outcomes is wide. A population survey of people aged 65 years that asked them how they perceived quality of life reported that they emphasised psychological characteristics (e.g. outlook on life), health and functional ability, social relationships, neighbourhood (e.g. safety, facilties, transport), having enough money and retaining their independence.[7]

On a day-to-day basis, quality of life on the ward may have to be based on subjective assessment, taking into account what the patient thinks, and his or her morale, ability to communicate, mental capacity, degree of incontinence and physical dependency. For example, a person with end-stage dementia who cannot recognise their loved ones can be assumed to have reached a stage where, to that person, the meaning of human life has deteriorated, and they therefore have a poor quality of life.

# Choosing a measure of health-related quality of life

When choosing a health-related quality-of-life measure, or a battery of measures, key questions to consider are whether a *generic* or *disease-specific* measure is needed, and whether this should be supplemented with more detailed *domain-specific* measures (e.g. depression scales) that are important to the aims of the study. The type of scale and domain-specific scales will vary according to the type of patient under study.

Generic measures usually tap social, psychological and physical areas of life. They are used for population health profiles and in order to make comparisons with other conditions (e.g. outcome of treatments for different conditions). The latter are useful when comparisons of the costs of treatments in relation to their benefits (outcomes) are required.

# Popular measurement scales

One of the most popular, concise generic measures is the Short Form 36-item Health Survey Questionnaire (SF-36).[8] This is also often used as a core component to facilitate comparisons across populations in disease-specific batteries of measures. These need to be interviewer administered to obtain the best item response rates among elderly people.[9] In the USA, a commonly used generic scale developed for use with elderly people is the Older Americans' Resources and Services Schedule (OARS), although the full instrument is lengthy.[10]

Because of the multiple morbidity that is often found in older people, and potential effects on physical functioning, emotional well-being and mental state, most investigators prefer to use a battery of pertinent domain-specific scales when evaluating the health status or health outcomes of elderly people. These may be used together with relevant disease-specific or generic measures, while bearing in mind the need to limit respondent fatigue. Popular domain-specific scales include Lawton's (1975) Philadelphia Geriatric Center

Morale Scale,[11] the Abbreviated Mental Test (AMT)[12] and the Geriatric Depression Scale (GDS).[13] A concise measure of anxiety and depression, which does not include somatic items and is therefore appropriate for use with older people, is the Hospital Anxiety and Depression Scale (HADS).[14] The Barthel Index[15] is often used to measure physical functioning, but this is only suitable for severely ill, institutionalised populations. It focuses on self-care at the expense of instrumental tasks of daily living (e.g. domestic tasks) and wider physical mobility. The functioning sub-section of the Older Americans' Resources and Services Schedule is superior to most scales for use with elderly people.

There is no consensus on recommended batteries of scales. More recently there has been an emphasis on also asking people to list themselves what areas of their life are most important or which have been most affected by their condition. Given that people will have different priorities in life (e.g. the ability to go up a flight of stairs is less important to someone who does not have stairs), these newer instruments provide the means by which individuality can be assessed scientifically. [16,17]

# Criteria for scale development and for selecting a scale

The criteria for measurement scales or batteries of scales are listed below.[18] When reviewing scales for use, potential users should check the scale's literature for information on each of these areas, and use an appropriate scale where this information is satisfactory.

## Conceptual and measurement model

The conceptual and empirical basis for combining multiple items into a single scale score(s) should be provided. Descriptive statistics for each scale should be provided by scale developers (frequencies, means, central tendency and dispersion, skewness and frequency of missing data), as should procedures for weighting and scoring.

## Reliability

The instrument should be free from random error and therefore homogenous in content (high correlations between items and tests of internal consistency). It should be reproducible over time (where changes in scores are not expected) and between raters at one point in time. Scale developers should provide a clear description of the methods used to test for reliability, by type of population, and information on the results of tests for reliability.

# Validity

This is the degree to which an instrument measures what it purports to measure. The scale developer should provide evidence that the content of the scale is appropriate and relevant to its intended use, that its construct is sound and that it correlates with measures with which it is theoretically expected to correlate, and that it correlates with a criterion measurement ('gold standard'). As with reliability, full details of the methods, samples and results of tests of validity should be provided by the developer.

# Responsiveness

This is the sensitivity of the instrument to true change (e.g. in the patient's condition). This is assessed in before–after studies of interventions and a comparison of scale scores. Assessment of responsiveness involves estimation of the effect size. This is an estimate of the magnitude of change in health status, and it translates the before–after changes into a standard unit of measurement. Scale developers should provide information on responsiveness from longitudinal study data on clearly defined populations.

# Interpretability

This is the degree to which meaning can be assigned to the scale's scores. It can be provided by comparative data on the distribution of scores in different populations and on the relationship of scores to clinically recognised conditions and outcomes (including predictive ability of the score in relation to death). The scale developer should provide details of the populations to whom the scale was administered and descriptive statistics.

# Burden

Respondent burden can be defined as the time, energy and other demands placed on the respondents during the completion of the instrument. Administrative burden is the demand placed on those who administer it. Developers should not place undue strain on the respondent during the completion of their instruments, and should provide information on average completion times, comprehension or reading levels required, interviewer training required, and the acceptability of the instrument (e.g. indicated by the level of missing data and refusal rates plus reasons).

# Alternative forms

These include all of the modes of administration of an instrument, such as self-completion, observer ratings, interviewer administered and computer-assisted completion. Evidence of reliability, validity, responsiveness, interpretability and burden should be provided for each form of the instrument.

# Cultural and language adaptations

The scale developer should provide information about the conceptual equivalence (equivalence of relevance and meaning of the same concepts) and linguistic equivalence (equivalence of question wording and meaning in the formulation of items, response choices) of the scale in the different languages and repeat the evaluations of its measurement properties (reliability, validity, responsiveness, interpretability and burden). The scale developer should provide evidence of the methods used to achieve equivalence (e.g. assessment within each cultural or language group to which the instrument will be applied, two forward translations from the source language by experienced translators and health status research, resulting in a pooled forward translation; backward translations to the source language resulting in a pooled translation; review of translations by lay and expert panels, with revisions and field testing to provide evidence of comparability and explanation of any differences).

These criteria should be used to evaluate the strengths and weaknesses of measurement instruments. A wide range of generic and disease-specific measurement scales were concisely reviewed by Bowling in 1995[9] and 1997.[19]

---

**Key points**

- People themselves are the best judges of an outcome of 'life worth living'.
- The only way to address an ethical dilemma about treatment is to ask the patient about their perception of their quality of life and their preferences.
- If the patient is not competent to answer this question, then ask their next of kin or carer who knows them best.

- In the ward setting, quality of life may have to be assessed after taking into account the views of the patient and their carers with regard to morale, their symptoms as well as their physical dependency, their mental capacity and whether they are incontinent.
- Although there is no consensus on the recommended battery of scales, commonly used instruments include Lawton's Philadelphia Geriatric Morale Scale, the Abbreviated Mental Test and the Geriatric Depression Scale.

# References

1  McNeil BJ, Weichselbaum R and Pauker SG (1978) Fallacy of the five-year survival in lung cancer. *NEJM*. **299**: 1397–401.

2  McNeil BJ, Weichselbaum R and Pauker SG (1981) Speech and survival: trade-offs between quality and quantity of life in laryngeal cancer. *NEJM*. **305**: 982–7.

3  Slevin ML, Stubbs L, Plant HJ *et al*. (1990) Attitudes to chemotherapy: comparing views of patients with cancer with those of doctors, nurses and the general public. *BMJ*. **300**: 1458–60.

4  Liddle J, Gilleard C and Neil A (1993) Elderly patients' and their relatives' views on CPR [letter]. *Lancet*, **342**: 1055.

5  Bowling A, Bond M, McClay M *et al*. (2001) Equity in access to exercise tolerance testing, coronary angiography, and coronary artery bypass grafting by age, sex and clinical indications. *Heart*. **85**: 680–6.

6  Walter PJ and Mohan R (1994) Health-related quality of life in octogenarians 5 years after coronary bypass surgery. *Qual Life Res*. **3**: 63.

7  Bowling A, Gabriel Z, Dykes J *et al*. (2003) Let's ask them: a national survey of definitions of quality of life and its enhancement among people aged 65 and over. *Int J Ageing Hum Dev*. **56**: 269–306.

8  Ware JE, Snow KK, Kosinski M and Gandek B (1993) *SF-36 Health Survey: manual and interpretation guide*. The Health Institute, New England Medical Center, Boston, MA.

9  Bowling A (1995) *Measuring Disease. A review of disease-specific quality-of-life measurement scales* (2e). Open University Press, Buckingham.

10  Fillenbaum GG and Smyer MA (1981) The development, validity and reliability of the OARS Multidimensional Functional Assessment Questionnaire. *J Gerontol*. **36**: 428–34.

11  Lawton MP (1975) The Philadelphia Geriatric Morale Scale: a revision. *J Gerontol*. **30**: 85–9.

12  Hodkinson HM (1972) Evaluation of a mental test score for assessment of mental impairment in the elderly. *Age Ageing*. **1**: 233–8.

13  Ysavage JA, Brink TL, Rose TL *et al*. (1983) Development and validation of a geriatric depression screening scale – a preliminary report. *J Psychiatr Res*. **17**: 37–49.

14 Zigmond AS and Snaith RP (1983) The Hospital Anxiety and Depression Scale. *Acta Psychiatr Scand.* **67**: 361–70.

15 Mahoney FI and Barthel DW (1965) Functional evaluation: the Barthel Index. *Md State Med J.* **14**: 61–5.

16 O'Boyle CA, McGee H, Hickey A *et al.* (1989) Reliability and validity of judgement analysis as a method for assessing quality of life. *Br J Clin Pharmacol.* **27**: 155.

17 Bowling A (1996) The effects of illness on quality of life: findings from a survey of households in Great Britain. *J Epidemiol Com Health.* **50**: 149–55.

18 Medical Outcomes Trust (1996) Source pages. In: *Products, Applications, Services. A resource directory for the health outcomes field.* Medical Outcomes Trust, Boston, MA.

19 Bowling A (1997) *Measuring Health. A review of quality-of-life measurement scales* (2e). Open University Press, Buckingham.

# Addendum

Recent judgement from the European Court of Human Rights (Glass v United Kingdom – Application No: 61827/00) stated that doctors/hospital authorities cannot override a relative's objection to the treatment of a disabled person without the authorisation by a court under the right to respect for private life, as guaranteed by Article 8 of the European Convention on Human Rights. This means that doctors must seek legal advice on withholding or withdrawing care if consensus cannot be reached between themselves and a patient's family.

# Index

Page numbers in italics refer to tables or case studies; *f.* refers to footnotes.